Top Tips to Best Birth
It's Your Baby
The Busy Woman's Guide
To a stress free pregnancy and birth

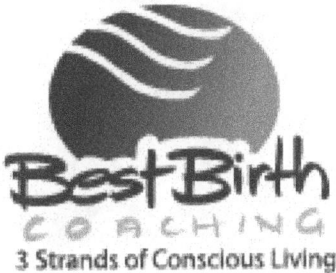

3 Strands of Conscious Living

ROSIE MCCAFFREY,
FOUNDER; BEST BIRTH COACHING,
REGISTERED NURSE, IYTA YOGA TEACHER, REIKI
MASTER, ADVANCED CERT NEURO EMOTIONAL
TECHNIQUE, MASTERS COUNSELLING

The busy woman's guide to a
stress free pregnancy and birth

Top Tips to
Best Birth

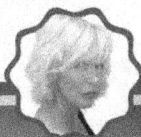

Rosie McCaffrey

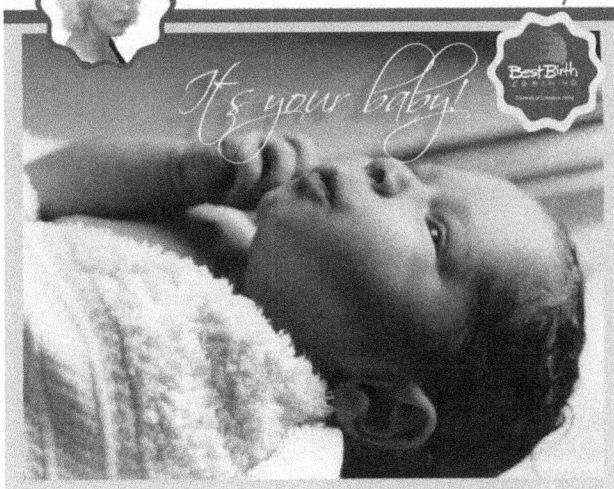

It's your baby!

Best Birth Coaching Top Tips for Best Birth
It's your Baby.

The busy woman's guide to a stress free pregnancy and birth.

Rosie McCaffrey, RN,
Master Social Health, IYTA

Disclaimer

The people and events described and depicted in this book are for educational purposes only. While every attempt has been made to verify the information provided in this book, the author assumes no responsibility for any errors, inaccuracies or omissions.

If advice regarding health or related matters is needed, the services of a qualified professional should be sought. The examples in this book will not guarantee that everyone or anyone else will achieve their desired results. His or her dedication, effort and motivation will determine each individual success. There are no guarantees that you will achieve your desired outcomes.

2013 by Rosie McCaffrey All Rights Reserved.

National Library of Australia Cataloguing-in-Publication entry

Author: McCaffrey, Rosie, author.

Title: Best birth : it's your baby the busy woman's guide to a stress free pregnancy and birth / Rosie McCaffrey.

ISBN: 9780992449407 (paperback)

Subjects: Pregnancy. Childbirth.

Dewey Number: 618.2

Published by Best Birth Coaching
Killarney Heights NSW 2087 Australia
Email. Bestbirth.com.au
For further information about orders: Phone +61 4 02847382

Testimonials

"I believe the book will be invaluable to both pregnant women and to those who teach them Yoga."

Debbie Hodges, Journalist, Pre natal IYTA Yoga Teacher and mother of two.

"Gold, gold, gold."

Lois Nethery, Ocean Acupuncture, former student with university degrees in psychology and Chinese medicine and mother of two.

"Highly endorsed"

by Mary-Louise Parkinson, Co-ordinator and Lecturer, IYTA Post graduate Diploma in Pre and Post Natal Yoga, former student and mother of two.

Dedication

This series, and all the work that comes from it is dedicated to my mother, who always encouraged me to "walk the road less travelled", and be, all I can be...

Best Birth Coaching Series

Best Birth Coaching is a series of books developed for wellness intervention for pregnancy, birth and beyond. Rosie McCaffrey shares her knowledge and experience for everyone concerned with pregnancy and birth. In a genre with many available titles, this book carves out a special niche and offers original content to soon-to-be mothers. By focusing on the emotional, social, and cultural aspects of pregnancy, this book is a strong supplement to the medical and anatomical information that pregnant women are inundated with.

Author Rosie McCaffrey

Rosie McCaffrey has been practicing yoga since the age of seven. She established one of the first prenatal yoga classes in Sydney and has sponsored and supported many of the leading prenatal teachers in the area. She has recent acute experience in this area of the medical world, and compassionately understands all of the complex pathways and processes for the women. She has received "high distinctions" for her ability to run "group" in completion of her master in counselling. She has a deep understanding in how women "cope" through the process of a traumatic birth experience with the completion of her thesis, and has an outstanding past history for coaching women through their pregnancy to have a "best birth" outcome for women and their families. She is highly skilled in her understanding of "energetics", and how these can be applied to support women in group and individual session. Rosie McCaffrey, as "Best Birth" has a continued passion, with 30 years of experience to promote the 'Best Birth" outcomes for women in our community.

EXCITING NEWS!

BestBirth coaching is taking technology and innovation to the next level in interactive book publishing.

Throughout this book you will see scanable QR codes that will allow you to watch, listen, learn, visit and download information relevant to the topics within this book.

Enjoy the experience!

All you need to do is use your tablet, iPhone, android smartphone or ipad QR scanner to scan the QR codes within the pages of this book to be redirected to the videos, opt-ins, downloads, audios and special offers. If you do not have an iPhone or ipad to scan the QR codes you can visit manually via your app store or Itunes to download a scanner.

Android QR Scanner App
:https://play.google.com/store/apps/details?id=me.scan.android.client

IPhone & Ipad QR Scanner App:
https://itunes.apple.com/en/app/qr-reader-for-iphone/id368494609?mt=8

To view welcome video from Rosie McCaffrey
http://www.bestbirth.com.au/book

Table of Contents

SCAN HERE FOR YOUR INTRODUCTORY VIDEO

ACKNOWLEDGEMENTS

As I reach the point of publishing my book, I am genuinely filled with humility and awe at the people who have touched my life. I hold the profound belief that every person we met affects us at some level. As we act out our lives how we are in the world, our being has a rippling effect in our interactions with each other. I for my part have faced up to my journey, with a willingness to engage with, and learn from, all that I come across. I have at times struggled with my own issues but I have remained on my path and I have reached the end of yet another chapter in my life, that of "the unpublished "author.

As I sit here now reflecting,I realize I have had an amazing story, starting with my family of origin, to whom I say thank you for your love and support. I apologize that I abandoned you physically to explore the greater world, but that is what I was taught by you to do. You know that you are always carried in my heart.

I say thank you to all my colleagues in the world of nursing and medicine. I have learnt something from all of you. Your commitment to gain knowledge and uphold exceptional standards of health care day in, day out is inspiring. Twenty-four hours a day, seven days a week we turn up to assist people through the traumatic events of peoples' lives. We do this to keep them safe when they can no longer do this for themselves. I am honored to say I have worked throughout the world, in different cultures, with teams of people who share the common goal of delivering the best for their patients. I have met so many inspiring people on this path, people who strive for continued excellence in what they deliver.

As a yogi, I have learned the art of strength, flexibility, non-judgment and compassion. A balanced approach. It has helped me build a foundation of values and beliefs that allow me to take courageous actions in my life. I have been privileged to study under many of the leading contemporary yogis and spiritual masters of the world and I say with gratitude "thank you" for the generosity with which you willingly shared your knowledge, supported me and gave me space to grow.

To all of my many "teachers", both academic and informal, in all the arts and sciences I have studied, I have learned something from every one of you, which I now share. Thank you.

To my ex-husband Angus, with whom I shared my life for twenty-five years, and for the relationship that allowed me to be a mother, I also thank you. We have two beautiful children who are now young adults whom we have nurtured and loved together. We did two things really well, and enjoyed the journey, the highs and the lows as a united front to support our children's growth. We had a common goal in creating our family, bringing two unique little beings into the world and raising them up to be all they can be. "Job well done Angus, thank you."

The most sublime emotions fill my heart at the thought of my children, as I look for words to describe it. Without the experience they have brought me, I would be ill prepared to write this book. In truth motherhood was not what I expected, for they were once part of me, they know what my heart sounds like on the inside and now they have grown up into wonderfully independent, capable and beautiful people. Naturally, they don't relate back to what they were as babies and toddlers. All the fun love and work that goes into them has passed. They are formed young adults now. Pride, awe, love respect and a lot of boundary setting is what comes to my mind in the form of words, but if there is a love that defines this world, it would be the love of a mother for her child, and my love of my children that creates the "why" in my life. "Thank you for being" is such an inadequate expression for what I feel towards you.

Lastly, to all the women who have trusted me to care for you and coach you on your journey, I say "thank you". It doesn't matter how much knowledge, wisdom and experience we collect on the journey if you are not open to learning, it cannot be shared. Your feedback on my approach to holding your space in your pregnancy has continually inspired me to keep going through the tough times. It is only on a shared journey that we can keep going.

Finally, to all the contemporary women out there, who through the process of motherhood face continual change at a pace which is unprecedented in our history, I salute you, for you are my inspiration and hope for the future.

Top tips to Best Birth

IT S YOUR BABY:

THE BUSY WOMEN'S GUIDE TO A STRESS-FREE PREGNANCY AND BIRTH

Welcome.

If you are reading this book, you are presumably going through what I have only experienced twice in my life, and yet both times it was an amazing experience, one with no equal. Every woman feels this each time they find out they are pregnant. The mystery of conceiving and finding out you are with child is the biggest shock to the psyche, even if it is a planned, wanted, well-loved and anticipated pregnancy. If you have received the news that you are pregnant your life and sense of self has already been imprinted and it will never be the same again, whatever the outcome. You are in a transition, and on a journey.

In our modern world with a limitless amount of information, expertise, and research, what is really helpful to draw upon as you navigate through this profound experience? It's really not to be missed with moments that are full of the most intense emotions you are going to experience in your life. Yet with so much advice out there, it can be a stressful, confusing and at times overwhelming.

My market research, from years of helping people in this area has shown me that the majority of women believe that "nothing can prepare you for birth", but I disagree. The women that do my courses state that they feel confident and excited about the process of birth. This is because they are ready. They used the time of pregnancy to prepare themselves for the biggest event in our lives.

How we each manage varies widely. Some people consume every piece of knowledge they can get their hands on, alter their lifestyles, become very precious about themselves and their baby, while other women cope by putting on blinkers, ignoring the obvious and miss some of the most spectacular moments in their lives. There is a whole spectrum of skills utilised to navigate this moment, where you sit on the scale is an individual response to a lifetime of learning and events. It's your pregnancy and you have to know yourself to know where you stand with it.

There is no right or wrong way; a contemporary woman is a busy person who is already multi -tasking in many different roles. Task rich, time poor, stressed, anxious, avoiding being overwhelmed by complacency or minimalizing the impact that pregnancy will have on her life and the fact that there is a whole team of experts out there that can manage your pregnancy for you. Through developing an understanding and insight into your pregnancy, you will be well on your way to a guilt- and stress-free pregnancy and birth.

In part one we discuss the issue of mental strength. Mental strength is as important as physical strength in pregnancy. With any journey you need to plan well to minimize stress. You need to know where you are at the start, know where it is you want to go, what you need to bring, and who your travelling companions will be, and of course you need a map and guide book. We will also be exploring some of the things you can do when things go wrong, break down or take a wrong turn so that you can get back on track and find the best birth outcome for you and your baby.

We will achieve this with some old school coaching for the contemporary woman in a friendly and personal way. Women have been birthing since the dawn of time and we are amazing creatures, but times, methods, attitudes and beliefs change and we must adapt to survive. We will be busting some common myths about the process of pregnancy and birth and developing some etiquette guidelines that suit you. Building confidence in yourself through practice and skill development so that you know you are doing the right thing for you and your baby.

In this book, the state or place of pregnancy will be viewed as paramount, to support the woman as she moves from a place where she is not a mother, to the place where she can effectively mother another complete human being she has conceived, grown and nurtured. This book is about the period of time, the inner journey, the knowledge and experience she has already formed, from the conception of her baby, to their shared birth event, and aims to privilege the process of pregnancy through the voice or views of the woman who is to become a mother.

The beauty of this book is that it is designed for busy women to meet your needs, by offering quick, concise, "take as much or as little as you like" style. Simply in the reading of the book you will join the journey. It is written in a reflective, friendly manner which provides you with easy to do exercises, case studies, and a proven method to map out your journey so that you have a very high chance of getting there – to a stress-free best birth outcome. Let's begin.

CHAPTER ONE –

VISION AND PURPOSE, WHY BUILD MENTAL STRENGTH

It is OK to say no

When we are pregnant, lots of people want to give us things and they are all packaged in different ways. Presents come in all shapes, sizes and forms. Some are wanted and some are not. We've been taught as girls to get excited about receiving gifts. Receive them with manners; open them with anticipation and give back a grateful response. On occasions these presents will be perfect, just what you wanted and you will use them every day. Why? Because the person who bought you the gift cared enough about you to pay attention, find out what it was you wanted the most, went out of their way to track it down,

wrap it up and give it to you. Why?
Because they cared, they are in a real
relationship with you and they want to
make you happy. Their payoff is that they
get to share the joy.

However, many people give a present
because it is what they want to receive.
They think about what will bring pleasure
to them, and assume it most bring
pleasure to you because they care about
you and perceive you to be the same.
This is called a projection. It's more about
how they want the world to look rather
than how you want the world to look. It's
more about what they want than what
you want. We often feign excitement in

accepting these gifts but are left having to use things in our daily lives that are not to our liking.

For most things, it's not important. Receiving money so you can purchase what you want instead of a gift is a sensible solution, but it misses the intimacy and pure joy of that perfect gift. Much the same can be said about your journey to birth, your relationship with your pregnancy and how you want to handle it. Giving your pregnancy a unique identity that both you and the world can relate to is important.

Your pregnancy is now part of you, but separate in that it is a stage or process that will end. This identity is only temporarily with you for nine months and in real time it will be gone and lost forever.

The word pregnant has a loaded connotation. You will be growing, changing and adapting quicker, faster and with a permanence that you have never encountered before. Some women have said that nothing can prepare you for birth but I would like to offer that nature has given us pregnancy to adjust our load. What we do with this gift is up to us. If we use the time to develop our mind, our awareness, as well as our body, being present in the process, we can begin to own our experience of it, which brings its own payoffs along the way.

Your pregnancy will be a unique chapter in your life, the consequences of which will stay with you forever. Each and every one is so different, yet every single person that walks the planet does so because a woman has been pregnant and successfully given birth. This contradiction in concepts is a wonderful thing. Pregnancy and birth is so unique yet so common. This concept alone is what gives so many professionals, who have worked in perinatal care for years, the ability to re-engage in their professional roles with fresh vigour and attitude every day. Nothing is more important to you than your pregnancy and this is all about you.

Myth # 1 Doctors are the experts and to be a good patient you must do what they say…

Doctors are professional people who specialise in a particular area of health care. They have undergone many years of specialist training, are peer reviewed and licensed by the health care system. They are the experts in their field and are capable of giving you professional advice. Nevertheless, they are not gods, and one of their responsibilities is to keep the patient informed for her own well-being and decision-making.

Hence, despite their medical expertise, they are not the expert on you, your relationships, your pregnancy or your family. *You* are, and doctors should do all they can to inform you, encourage you, care for you and keep you safe. When you are unable to do this for yourself they will step in through their legal obligations and take over for you, but only in an extreme emergency situation, as we will explore later in the book.

Based upon my experience and research in perinatal care, the majority of pain in a situation is expressed through having a lack of knowledge of events. It is this lack of knowledge in the moment that is so painful because you are unable to make a decision and move forward, forced to take responsibility for a situation and maybe left with regret about your actions. Let me introduce you to Michelle, who volunteered as a research candidate for my thesis.

Case study

Michelle is a 35-year-old, highly intelligent, happily married woman with a university education and professional career, one involving a big job. She is in a loving, caring and supportive relationship with her partner. If anything, it was Michelle who offered the support in her relationship as she is a strong, capable young woman who was able to be in control. Michelle came from a middle class home and as a result of her father's occupation her family had moved through four continents as she was growing up. She had settled in Australia, where she created a life she loved.

Michelle -"*Oh I always knew I wanted to become a mother and have children and I think it was kind of, it was the right time for us. It's never, as you probably know, never a perfect time because there's always all these things that you would love to do but it was a really, it was a good time and we fell pregnant quicker than I anticipated so at first I think we were like, "oh well, oh my God," but it was a good time and it was planned and everything like that. OK, well I'll probably start with how it all happened until then I was really good, I was exactly as I was now, no issues everyone kept telling me like yeah, low*

risk pregnancy, everything was good

Rosie – What expectations did you hold

for your first pregnancy and birth?

Michelle – *"I know there are a lot of birth*

related questions, I don't reasonably

have any because the birth happened so

early like before I'd even attended any

classes, before I'd read anything on birth

so I really had no expectations at all! I

hadn't even thought about it so I can't

tell you to much about that just because

yeah I really, I hadn't even gotten there

and um, pregnancy I just oh I just I don't

know, I just because I was pretty, like fit

and healthy and everyone kept telling

me that, the pregnancy and everything

was good. I think I just assumed I would just lead my normal life more or less until I, until the baby arrived. I was planning to go onto maternity leave pretty early at maybe thirty, thirty-one weeks.

Michelle was booked into a private hospital that had a large maternity department with a great reputation. She was not anticipating any complications and was completely unprepared when her waters broke at twenty-three weeks. Michelle – *"I didn't have a clue! What it was going to be like or how it could look, like I just hadn't read anything about it or even heard anything about it or thought about it and yes... someone should have just said to me 'you just lie there try not to stress' and hopefully it would really have been better."*

Michelle's story is a very complex one, which is one of the reasons I chose it. It involves ethical, legal, medical and personal consequences and implications. This reflects some of the issues that may cause you worry, but had Michelle been more informed about her story and her process, she may have been able to make the event slightly less painful because she was aware of her pregnancy and understood what her bottom line was. Taking ownership of your pregnancy is the best way to get what you want, your best birth outcome. We will be covering how to do this later in the book. You will develop psychological flexibility and strength. By understanding what you look at, how you position yourself and what you chose to ignore, is like receiving a present for life. When you look at it like this, why would you not want to open up the box and find out what's inside?

Myth #1
Busted!

Doctors like their patients to be informed because it makes hard decisions at the time of birth more achievable for everyone. Being a good patient nowadays is being an *informed* patient. Since the late 1970's, much work has been done in our society to educate all women on the ins and outs of pregnancy to improve birth outcomes for our women and our society in general.

This has widely been achieved through birth preparation and parenting classes being made available through maternity units. These classes offer scientific and medical information about the process of pregnancy and birth, group viewing of a birth through vaginal delivery and caesarean section, discussion about available interventions, what might be used for pain relief and emergency situations, and most importantly, it gives you an opportunity to see the place where you will give birth, meet the staff who may be caring for you and have the opportunity to have your questions answered and become familiar with the strangeness of the environment.

The increasing complexity of medical techniques have fuelled the misconception that a high intervention birth is the safest process and by implication is the *normal* process. Our paradigms or ways of looking or acting upon birth are changing. Understanding what our values and beliefs are is an important aspect of personal growth for women on their journey through to motherhood, to accept and accommodate the best birth outcome.

The journey of pregnancy is also a series of yes and no decisions that *you* will have to make. It takes courage to say no, but sometimes, for your own sake, you just have to. We all want to feel good about ourselves, yet some situations lead us to a place where we don't. Events in the moment don't always go the way we might like them to. Sometimes how we feel about ourselves depends on how we let other people affect us. Saying yes when you would rather say no can lead to stress, aches and pains, body tension and sleepless nights.

Here are a few tips on how to gracefully decline things you don't want. Remember you are saying no to the request, not the person. Saying no doesn't mean you are rejecting that person, or that you don't like them. Stay calm, polite and be honest. Indecision and a delayed refusal are more apt to upset someone than an immediate no.

If it is appropriate, give a brief and genuine refusal without opening up the discussion for future negotiation. Do not apologize. Be direct and succinct. "No thank you." If you genuinely want to meet the request at another time, take a rain check, acknowledge the other person's request, reflect the content and feeling, but add an assertive refusal.

What makes us want to say yes or no?

The reason we are able to hold preferences and make decisions is because we understand our values and beliefs. We all have an internalized system of values and beliefs that we have developed throughout our lives, guiding our actions and shaping our behaviour. However, it's important to distinguish between values and beliefs.

Values

Our values are things that we deem important and can include concepts like safety, equality, respect, education, effort, perseverance, trust, etc. Our values are largely tailored to our own individual character and they affect us at a deep subconscious level. Every decision we make is based on our values, which we use either as avoidance, to move away from a situation, or for aspiration, to move towards what we want. Our values help us to resolve hidden conflicts, remove stresses and give us a firm direction in life. Ultimately they are important motivational tools for helping you move towards solutions and away from problems.

Beliefs

Our beliefs, on the other hand, are assumptions that we make about the world. Beliefs generally fall into two categories, empowering beliefs and limiting beliefs.

They grow from what we see, hear, experience, read and think about and they apply not only to how we see ourselves but also how we see other people and how we believe other people see us. We tend not to question our beliefs because we are so certain about them, especially those deep-seated beliefs that stem from childhood.

However, our beliefs can be changed or turned round by the re-remembering of events to thicken thin scripts, self-talk or ideas about ourselves. Empowering beliefs help us to confidently make changes. We use our empowering beliefs to make decisions in what can often be an ambiguous world. Limiting beliefs do the exact opposite and keep us rooted in particular problem or positions. Our limiting beliefs are often based on assumptions that are not true, and if you spend a lot of time saying that you can't do something, often, that's exactly what will happen – a 'self-fulfilling prophecy' of sorts originating from negative thinking.

A belief is said to communicate directly with the intelligence of our heart, as the truths contained in such communication cannot be expressed by words. This is an emotional response to a thought or concept.

The meaning of metaphors used in this book

A metaphor is a story that safely allows you to explore your underlying world view and explore the values that shapes your understanding of a situation. Metaphors will be used throughout this book to gives you a framework to explore your identity of pregnancy and motherhood and will facilitate you to make meaning of the process as it changes. They are cognitively important and help define our thoughts and actions. Metaphors will be used in context, to link the stories of events, according to your plot or pattern to assist you in understanding your personal meaning, who you are now, and assist you on your journey in how you become a mother.

Quick Quizzes – How to approach them

As we go through the activities, you are invited to create your child's most inspiring bedtime story for the first few years of their lives. Please tell me if I'm wrong, but my children loved nothing more than their bedtime story being all about them. I recorded the journey of my pregnancy as a reflective style journal, with photos and short stories of what I did, what they did, and what we did together. There are many pre-printed journals or pregnancy dairies you can purchase, or you can just get an A4 folder, cover it and keep your souvenirs as you like.

I am fairly confident that you feel like you already know the answers to some of the quizzes. You've done tests like these many times before. It's great that you know what you know, and building your confidence in your knowledge as you move towards your birth is one of the key aims of this book. However, extra practice can always benefit you and your baby. So grab a piece of paper and some coloured pens, let your own inner child out as you practice playfulness with your thoughts, ideas and expression of communications for your baby.

Centering techniques

—

click this link to listen

Through out the book are various techniques to help you stay focused and relaxed. As you listen to my voice it will assist you with your read of my book, as it will allow you to access my style of presentation. I hope you enjoy it.

Quick quiz # 1 – finding your values

Values are simply a reflection of who you are and how you live your life. They are not morals, or principles but a reflection of how you chose to be. They are the desired qualities that give meaning to your life, and as such, they are essential to satisfaction, fulfilment and a less stressed lifestyle!

Below is a list of values. Circle the ten values that are most important to you based on your first instinctive response. Then cross out five – leaving the five values that you simply could not live without. Rank them in order of importance:

achievement, adventure, beauty, being free, being generous, charity, comfort, community, creativity, dignity, discovery, fame, family, growth, happiness, health, honesty, honour, humility, independence, individuality, integrity, intimacy, kindness, knowledge, leadership, learning, living a legend, leisure, life partner, love,

making a difference,

parenting, passion,

patriotism, peace, physical

activity, power, security,

seeing the world, self –

discipline, self- esteem,

service, simplicity,

spirituality, strengths,

success, time alone, truth,

using my talents, wealth

Journal activity – Write your mission statement

Think about your answers. In what ways do they impact your life? Write a letter or story or draw a picture for your baby, identifying how these values will influence them. What your hopes and dreams of the future will look like using these values. Your children won't be judging the quality of your work; they will simply be lapping up your attention.

To close this chapter, I will offer you a bedtime story taken from "Natural Brilliance" by Paul R. Scheel. It is a story for your conscious mind, inner child and a parable for your inner self. You may feel odd reading to your belly, but just know, someone is listening, and later, when you see that face, and when you see the delight in a familiar story, you'll know why it was a good thing to do.

The stretch stitch – a parable as told by Dr Paul Scheele

Once upon a time, there was a wise old seamstress whose business had flourished for decades. She owned a large shop, staffed by men and women, young and young at heart. The employees enjoyed a committed partnership of talents, knowledge and creative ideas.

One day, another business owner approached the seamstress and asked to what she attributed her success. She replied, "Our success is found in the lesson of the stretch stitch."

"Most of our work of joining two pieces of fabric together involves sowing a straight stitch to form a seam," the seamstress explained. "Most of the time it holds just fine, but it can break because it is brittle, ridged, and linear. If it breaks, it unravels. And that would be a problem right here," she said grabbing the man's sleeve and pointing to the seam between the sleeve and shoulder, "your sleeve would fall right to the floor, wouldn't it?"

"At a place like this, this place called 'on the bias', we need something different." Pointing her finger at the visitor's chest and winking, she added "and you have a bias for succeeding in business, don't you?"

The seamstress lowered her voice to a hoarse whisper to make sure the man listened carefully, and said "the most remarkable stitch is a simple one that takes two stitches forward and one stitch back. It is both strong and flexible – more so than any other. This stitch teaches all who are ready to succeed."

She leaned forward with a meaningful gaze and a twinkle in her eyes and continued, "Are you willing to take a step back with every few steps forward? Notice your progress. Learn from where you come from and look to where you are going. You will soon develop remarkable personal strength and flexibility. With these valuable resources you will succeed in any life endeavour."

CHAPTER 2 –

CREATING YOUR PROFILE

Bringing clarity into your picture

Being pregnant is both beautiful and scary. Physically and emotionally, we are in a vulnerable place. So much is going to change in your life, and you have to get through the birth yet! That is a normal part of the reaction, but how you deal with these challenges has great implications for you and your baby. It is the rite of passage into motherhood and like all arduous times in our life, both excitement and fear colour the process. Mental strength, while often overlooked, is what will empower you over that finish line.

How to Develop Mental Strengths

First off, it helps to know exactly what mental strength is. The definition that I like to use is that it's the ability to will oneself through less-than-ideal situations and conditions. Mental strength is typically not something you're born with, but rather, something that is developed by regularly operating outside of your comfort zone

Take this illustration for example...

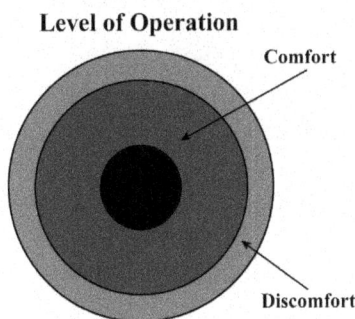

69

The centre circle represents you and your pregnancy, and the purple area is your present level of comfort. No extra amount of effort is required to stay there. This is your safe haven, your bad habits, those day-to-day ruts, your place of predictability and familiarity. In short, your level of comfort.

But now you're pregnant and encountering immense changes, changes which are only going to become more pronounced. Welcome to the red area. The red area beyond this circle represents your area of discomfort. This is the area in which you know you could operate if required to, but it's difficult and most people choose not to. This is one reason so many women chose not to prepare for birth appropriately. The process of pregnancy will place you both physically and emotional in this zone a lot of the time.

However, when you purposely choose to step just outside of your comfort zone, something interesting happens. With time, this larger area will become your new comfort zone and what was previously difficult now becomes easier — giving you a new and broader perspective on what your limitations are. You become a bigger person. Then, the whole cycle repeats itself, from birth as you progress to motherhood.

Expanding Your Comfort Zone

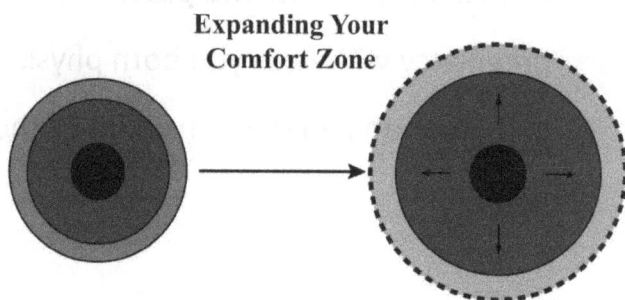

What this means is that now's the time to prepare for tough times ahead. Those times are coming! Your level of fitness or current age are inconsequential, since you can make the choice to go beyond your present level of comfort — ideally on a day-to-day basis.

Contemporary woman is very capable of higher order, awareness thinking, and thus you can learn skills to overcome your fears and limiting self-beliefs. In this book you can identify self-limiting beliefs and resulting patterns of behaviours that keep you from your goal – a best birth outcome.

Journal activity

Add a mental strengths segment to your journal.
Basically, record on a daily basis the things that
change. Note the things that take you out of your
comfort zone due to your pregnancy and you
manage anyway.

As you do so, you'll be able to look back and see
the progress you've made and what used to be
uncomfortable and difficult becomes
comfortable and easy. These can be easily
divided up into concepts and actions which
involve your normal activities for daily living or
'ADL's.'

Concepts are ideas that you have to change, like
being aware that people, even complete

strangers, now treat you differently as they see your baby bump develop, to having to experience examinations and blood tests that you normally wouldn't consent to. Diet, exercise, sleep and your choice of clothing all change. Notice what you like and don't like and remember to record it all with lots of photos. Your baby will love it.

Each time you make a choice to go beyond your comfort zone, you build up a reserve of mental strength. Each time you choose the easier path, you diminish that capacity. As you build mental strength, you will be able to call upon that reserve during your delivery — and overcome your limiting beliefs.

Myth # 2 - If you focus only on the positive, only good things will happen – She'll be right!

This is not a New Age book. Rather, its content is based on a combination of ancient wisdom and modern practice, accumulated over many years of experience. It emphasises events in relation to an internal world and an external world – how you see things and how others see you, in context to the events.

Sometimes, we need to look at our uncomfortable feelings in metaphoric terms, called shadow, the darkness to bring forth the light. Accepting our shadow can help us balance the polarity between our conscious and personal unconscious awareness. To quote astronaut Chris Hadfield, who has inspired a new generation to explore the unknown, to have a successful mission you must plan for the unknown and unexpected. "Once you've been around the world 2500 times like I have, you see that the world is really just a spaceship, and everybody is a crew member, we're not just all passengers". Chris is urging each person to take responsibility in their life; understanding your values and beliefs will give you direction for where you want to go and also, what role or position you want to take.

Psychologist Carl Jung originally coined the term 'shadow,' which is, according to the Longman Dictionary of Psychology and Psychiatry, an "accordant archetype that represents instincts inherited from lower organisms, manly sexual and aggressive instincts, which tend to be unacceptable to the conscious and therefore repressed into the personal

unconscious where they may form
complexes."

Shadow is that portion of self that we fail
to bring to conscious awareness and is
formed in a parallel fashion to the
development of our ego. In life we are
constantly viewing the world through an
overlay of our emotional reality, editing
what fits into our image of ourselves.
More often than not, that which does not
fit into our ideal model is moved into the
shadow part of our personal unconscious.
Jung gave great importance to the
concept of integrating the shadow into
our conscious and felt it was necessary to
do so in order to reach a healthy sense of

self-realisation. Jung stated, "Realisation of shadow is an eminently practical problem which should not be twisted into an intellectual activity, for it has far more meaning of a suffering and a passion that implicates the whole person."

As the process of conception is primarily a sexual act, both physically and conceptually, through our identification as female it is often taboo and repressed information that needs to be looked at. This can be difficult and embarrassing, as it is our most private and personal parts of ourselves that are being exposed. We are at our most vulnerable and safety is always an issue. You need to know that you are safe and develop confidence in taking the right steps for you. You will be the person that benefits the most and you must know how to access further help if you need it. Nothing is so awful that you can't talk with someone about it.

Free support services

In North America crisis pregnancy centers (CPC), sometimes called a pregnancy resource center (PRC), are a not for profit organization established to assist pregnant women generally with counseling related issues to abortion, pregnancy, and childbirth, and some may also offer additional non-medical services such as financial assistance, child-rearing resources, and adoption referrals. CPCs that qualify may also provide pregnancy testing, sonograms, and other services; however, the vast majority are not licensed and provide no medical services. As there are over 2,500 CPR's it is best to source the contact details locally, in your area. Pregnancy Counseling Australia provides a safe and confidential environment for callers to discuss their pregnancy concerns on the 24/7 line 1300 737 732. At any time of the day or night, from anywhere in Australia, you will be able to speak to a compassionate, non-judgmental counselor who understands your feelings and concerns. Experienced counselors connect callers with resources and appropriate services, where further assistance is required.

The UK provides a service called care confidential. This service provides confidential advice and support for anyone regardless of their age, beliefs, background, gender or circumstances. The service is provided by highly trained and experienced counselors who have been working with women and their partners who face concerns in the area of pregnancy, birth and loss. They can be contacted by UK residence on 0300 4000 999 if you live in the United Kingdom.

Quick Quiz 2 – Recognising strengths in weaknesses

Looking at the characteristic

strengths or qualities below pick as

many as you like that you believe describe you. List them down and now sort them into order through your priorities. Then cross out two. Keep doing this until you only have a list of your five core values.

Love, Performance, Achieving, Outstanding, Action orientated, Appreciation, Belief, Neat, Benevolent, Careful, Loyal, Clean, Cautious, Malleable, Credible, Daring, Mastery, Dedicated, Dependable, Memorable, Opportunity,

Determined, Openness,

Durable, Energetic, Original,

Enthusiastic, Personable,

Ethical, Merciful, Equality,

Neighbourly, Unity, Excellence,

Obedience, Faithful,

Perseverance, Fearless, Purity,

Noble, Sturdy, Finesse,

Learning, Forgiveness,

Kindness, Formidable, Valiant,

Togetherness, Stability,

Nurturing, Free-thinking,

Persistent, Fresh Fun, Gallant,

Resourceful, Practical,

Generous, Meaningful,

Genuine, Good, Objective,

Planning, Tough, Yes minded,

Gracious, Economical, Just,

Professionalism, Strengths, Zen,

Happy, Youthful, Truth,

Knowledge, Helpful, Optimistic,

Honesty, Lasting, Honourable,

Hope, Reserved, Imagination,

Politeness, Organization,

Immovable, Information,

Integrity, Intelligence, Joy,

Methodical, Analytical,

Principled, Orderly, Fair,

Vigorous, Conserving, Thorough, Flexible, Open to change, Virtuous, Experimenter, Curious, Vigilant, Adaptable, Tolerant, Team player, Wisdom

Journal activity

Design a symbol

Think about why these are important to you, and how your choices are going to effect your life, your baby and your family. You are going to have to practice dealing with conflicting values. Design a symbol, or draw a picture that reflects where you are at the moment and label it. Put as much detail in as you can. I have included one of mine from the past to assist you in visualizing the task. This symbol helped me gain strength when I needed to create massive amounts of change in my life.

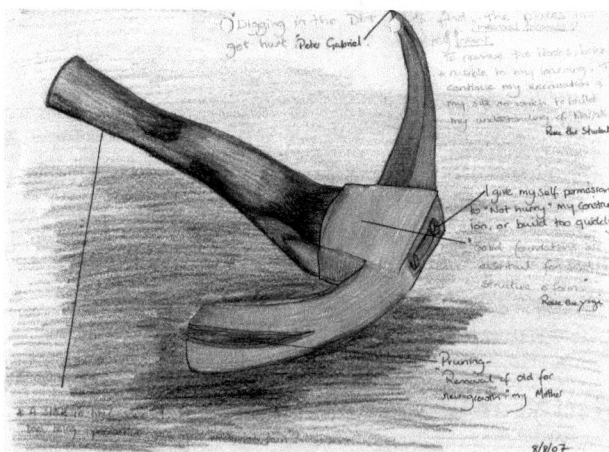

Quick Quiz 3 – Plotting Your Course

What are you bringing into your pregnancy with you? Use this link to plot out your pattern to see where you stand and how your values may shape your world. Notice any areas that are harder for you to map. Place an X in the line closest to your response.

What is your identity and how is it constructed?

The self is made up of many unfixed identities that are in a continual process of change. Through encounters with similarities and differences within other people, ideas, and places, we are able to understand ourselves and become more centered.

Quick quiz # 4 – How many identities do you already have

Labels are names we give to certain roles in our lives that can be limiting through design and association. Map out the roles that you have held in your life. You can subdivide categories to as much detail as you like. This is a really interesting exercise and shows just how many roles, responsibilities and how much life you have already experienced. To help you get going, here is an example of some of mine.

House keeper	Mother	Professional	Social
Traveller	Daughter	ICU Nurse	Coffee drinker
Writer	Cousin	Yoga teacher	Cinema goer
NICU nurse	Sister	Student	Party girl
Divorced	Cyclist	Yogi	Therapist
Community nurse	Wife	Counsellor	Friend

Identity grid
**Print out this sheet and fill all the roles you have held in your life.
Add it to your journal**

Identity is constructed through relationship, so getting to know your pregnancy is important. The process of identifying ourselves involves determining if others are like us or not like us, or being the same or different. We identify ourselves and are identified by others according to dichotomous logic. This means binary pairs such as male/female, person without child/mother, etc. These categories are who we are; they are real and culturally evident, but not natural, they are learned.

This ever-changing phenomenon of identity can be observed in a contextual instance. Meaning is produced from the binary pairs, from which our modern identities emerge. Even though we form our identities through comparing ourselves to others through different relationships, it allows us to form the most unique individual that we can be. We use similarities and difference within gender and sexuality to construct our identities and form vibrant, distinctive, and inquisitive individuals. There are very few true individuals. We are individuals only if we can think for ourselves and do not cling to other people's wishes and onto norms that are not always good.

Stress arises when we have conflicting values associated with our different roles or identities. I'm sure you may have experienced this already. Being pregnant will be affecting some of your current roles. Tiredness, nausea, frequency of passing water, food cravings, cramps, medical appointments, change in family commitments are among the common complaints of pregnancy.

Case study

Knowing where you are vulnerable is a very important tool in keeping yourself safe - physically and emotionally. To understand how conflicting values can affect our pregnancy, let's apply this to Michelle, our case study.

Michelle – "I was very, very busy at work [and it] was probably stressful as well, it was just unpleasant, just lots of people whining and complaining because they don't have anyone else to complain at. I was feeling really uncomfortable, thinking something's not right! But you know, I just didn't know what it was."

Michelle's professional and social success had left her with little time to reflect on her pregnancy. She wasn't the sort of person that was into *"soft music and candles stuff"*. However Michelle did have some great, proven resiliency skills that allowed her to manage as her son was born at 24 weeks and three days. *"I just focused, I pulled myself together and I just focused on what had to be done!"* Michelle was out of her comfort zone in all areas, but she was able to take tried and tested skills from her professional role and adapt herself to deal with this emergency.

*Michelle - **"then all of a sudden I just sort of felt this fluid coming out of me and went to the toilet and it just came gushing out, and I said to myself "OK so something's not right!***

"Then of the whole experience, I still think that was probably the worst part, it was like 23 weeks plus a few days and nobody knew what to do I think! I think my obstetrician was somehow secretly hoping I'd just start labour and it would all come out."

"I just developed this back pain and went into labour. It took me a long time to realise because of like, I didn't have a clue of what it was like or how it could look like.I don't know, your body sort of like wants to get it out, but you don't want it to come out . . . but at some stage I was just feeling miserable and something. I sort of wanted someone to get that - then he was born and after that it was pretty, it was just like a numbness more than anything."

Myth # 2 busted !

As you may have noticed in some of the examples, building your mental strength goes hand in hand with building your physical strength. Both of these are crucial when it comes to survival. Take this time to understand any conflicting values you may have through the many different roles you have to perform in your already busy life. Recognise the role that guilt may also play. Giving to others without taking care of yourself is an act of self-sabotage, but such self-denial, regardless of the cause, is always undermining and causes resentment and pain. Recognise whether or not this really is a problem for you and does it lie within your ability to change it. If you don't want to be an ostrich, what do you want to be? It is your pregnancy, what do you want to do with the time?

Ten minute relaxation technique

< click to hear

Enjoy

Bed time stories-
Sean Roach and the
Catapult team

Every morning on the Serengeti plains of

Africa...

A gazelle wakes up.

It *knows* from the moment it wakes that

it must run faster than the fastest lion...

Otherwise it WILL be killed!

Every morning on the same plains, a lion

wakes up.

It *knows* from the moment it wakes, that

it must outrun the slowest gazelle...

Or it WILL starve to death!

The wider moral to this story is, it doesn't matter whether you are a lion or a gazelle...

When the sun comes up on the plains...

You had BETTER get to running!

....

(So this is a cool little story, but what's it got to do with success principles and you?)

I'm glad you asked...

You see, whether you believe it or not, you have a choice about how you live your life...

Just like the gazelle you could choose to wake up each morning and be motivated by external factors.

Although you probably don't have a lion chasing you... maybe you rely on your boss, your partner, your teacher, your university lecturer, or *the law!*

(Take your pick)

BUT...

When you allow yourself to be dictated-to by the outside world, the only way you'll ever make progress towards *anything* is by being chased...

Meaning success comes in 'fits and spurts'.

(Think of a gazelle running from the lion, and then stopping to resume eating when the stimulus is removed)

We know a lot of people like this, right?

On the other hand, the lion.

She is internally motivated by hunger… the challenge of the hunt… and the thrill of the kill!

The lion understands that she can make a kill only about once in every five outings, and waiting in the grass… just a short distance away, looking on, are her hungry cubs.

A missed gazelle means she must return to the hunt immediately… failure is not an option!

The lion is a 'cause' in the world… not an 'effect'.

You might know people like the lion. They're the leaders of society, the wealthy or soon-to-be-wealthy, and the high-achievers of this world.

Heck! The very fact you are reading this probably makes you a lion...

What I'd like you to take from this story though, is the fact that (unlike the real lion and gazelle) you have the choice about whether you want to be...

Internally-motivated (success, wealth, happiness, purpose)

Or Externally-motivated (stress, fear, anxiety, mediocrity)

...The question is which do you choose?

To your success

Chapter Three –

What's stress got to do with it?

Stress

A clinical definition of stress is when environmental demands, both internal or external; real or imagined, tax or exceed the adaptive capacity of an organism, resulting in psychological and biological changes that may place persons at risk for disease. In my experience of the medical world stress first became a buzzword in the Eighties. It was spoken about in terms of being a "future" event. It was painted in black and dire terms and I made a commitment to myself that I wasn't going to meet it, if I had a choice. This decision set me on a lifelong path of learning. Predictions of overcrowded cities in Europe and a polluted planet left an indelible imprint on my mind and I committed myself to travel the world to see it before it was spoilt and to emigrate to Australia for a healthier, outdoors lifestyle and positive-she'll-be-right attitude.

Having lived through the social changes of the Nineties and turn of the millennium, stress now appears to be endemic. As much as I tried to avoid stress by leaving my job as an intensive care nurse to become a full time yoga teacher, therapist and counsellor, I still meet it.

This may have something to do with my own conflicting values of security and adventure, where my pendulum swings and my belief that life should be lived to its fullest. But my journey has allowed me to develop an interesting relationship with stress, and I have learnt how to manage it as a companion in life. Feeling stressed may feel like it's perfectly normal, especially when you're pregnant.

You are constantly living in the outer edge of your comfort zone with so much change. But it's also exciting. You might notice that sometimes being "stressed-out" motivates you to focus and organise yourself. It is, after all, a physiological response that excites the brain to action.

It is also necessary to understand that there is a distinction between acute and chronic stress. Acute stress results in a stress that is short lived because an effective resolution to the threat is achieved. However, chronic stress is of a longer duration and an effective resolution to the situation cannot be found in the immediate environment.

As a general rule, we try to find strategies to resolve our stress in one of two ways. First are problem focused strategies, or first order changes. These are aimed at changing the stressful situation outside of ourself. This refers to your efforts to alter the environment to meet your needs and includes beliefs that the reoccurrence or outcomes of a stressful event are subject to personal control.

Emotion-focused strategies, or second order change, are used to reduce the psychological tension, inside yourself or secondary control cognition. This describes a process where your sense of self changes to accommodate the environment and may include ascribing a purpose to your change or redefining the experience as beneficial.

Myth # 3 - Stress is good for you!

Stress is a burst of energy that basically advises you on what to do. In small doses, stress has many advantages. For instance, stress can help you meet daily challenges and motivates you to reach your goals. In fact, stress can help you accomplish tasks more efficiently. It can even boost memory.

Stress is also a vital warning system, producing the fight-or-flight response. When the brain perceives some kind of threat or danger, it starts flooding the body with chemicals like adrenaline, noradrenaline and cortisol. This creates a variety of reactions such as an increase in blood pressure and heart rate, so that more oxygenated blood is pumped into the muscles for a quick response action.

In addition, there are various health benefits associated with a little bit of stress. Some researchers believe that some stress can help to fortify the immune system, protecting your body from infection, and even improve recovery from surgery.

All things in moderation!

Therefore, stress is key for survival, but too much stress can be detrimental. Emotional stress that stays around for weeks or months can weaken the immune system and cause high blood pressure, fatigue, depression, anxiety and even heart disease, to name a few. Stressful events that are too big become traumatic, as the mind isn't able to process them.

It may be tough to tell whether you're experiencing perceived good or bad stress, but there are important benchmarks that you can look at to help point the way.

Busy women in busy times push through so much to get the job done, but we need to distinguish between stress and stimulation. Having deadlines, setting priorities, and pushing yourself to perform at capacity is stimulating. However these behaviors can lead to negative health outcomes when the demand and threat substantially tax or overwhelm your capacity to respond.

Stress is when you're anxious, upset, or frustrated, which dramatically reduce your ability to perform. People who get things done under stress are succeeding in spite of their stress, not because of it. They have developed coping strategies or resilience.

Case study

Michelle gives us great insight into how she deals with stress.

Rosie - So I'm just going to start by asking you the first question. If I could ask you what stress looks like for you?

Michelle – *"Um yeah I've just been thinking about it... um generally for me, I don't know, I thrive when I'm really busy so I wouldn't really call that stress. Stress for me is more, probably more anxiety sort of related on your stomach, sort of cramps up a bit I see that more, as stress. If I'm really busy and if I have lots on, I don't see it, like if stress is a negative thing I um don't see the stress, although it probably is a bit stressed because I tend to pack everything full and I, but I but for me stress is probably more yeah like anxiety, worry, I think that's more stressful..."*

Rosie – And is there anywhere that you feel that in your body?

Michelle – *"Um no not really. Just, sometimes I get really - in you know some situations when your stomach just cramps up - I would call that more stress. I lose weight if I'm stressed, of course you obviously only know that afterwards (laugh)."*

Rosie – So it's not really something that you're conscious of?

Michelle – *"No."*

Rosie – But later you might look back and notice you've lost weight. What other things might you notice?

Michelle – *"I really don't know, I've never, I've just never perceived stress as anything really like negative, where people say "I'm stressed, I've got so many appointments and so many things on". I just, you know it doesn't really bother me generally"*

Rosie – "And you still sleep and everything?"

Michelle- *"It depends what it is like. If I just have a lot on - yeah then sometimes work back then that would affect me, if you've got a bit too much on, if I, then I didn't know how to solve something or sort something out it would sometimes affect my sleep but then I generally, at some stage - I adopted that thing, like I have a pad next to my bed and if I just wrote things down then in the morning, you know how you look it and you're like 'it's ridiculous, it's really not worth losing sleep.' So yeah, that worked quite well."*

Michelle's unawareness of factors in her life had induced a stress response that pervaded her system. She was unaware of it until after the event, because she had convinced herself she could manage without looking at the shadow information which was available to her. This had a really negative affect on her pregnancy outcome, as we will explore in the next chapter. Michelle's way of coping was simply "not to look at it," which in the end, may have tripped her up a bit.

Myth #3 Busted!

Dr. Hans Selye, the reported founder of the modern stress concept, originally created this myth. Selye found that activities that exhort you like sex and sports also produced a surge in stress information substances, like birth, so he promoted the idea of good stress. However research has since shown that stress contributes to 75% to 90% of medical conditions, including the six leading causes of death. Stimulation is good for you - Stress is not.

Stress is often associated with bad experiences, so you might think it would bias your thinking in a negative direction. However, when people are put under stress, they begin paying more attention to positive information. Hope plays an important role in our appraisal systems, and we find it easier to cope if we position our self to see the positive in things, however, if you're not aware of this tendency and don't compensate for it, you might make some decisions you may later regret

In Summary

The physiological stress response has the goal of maintaining homeostasis, or normal functioning within your body. We normally cope by resolving the threat through problem solving or adapting ourselves. We can either try to change the outside world, where we have the baby, the style of birth, or we can change ourselves, understanding how to breath, position ourselves and build mental strength, or we may do both. Neither is the absolute right choice and both approaches are helpful. There is no correct formula; it comes down to what you want and how you manage it.

Quick quiz # 5 – wheel of life stress ball App

So lets start by breaking this down into bite size pieces. The eight sections in the wheel of life will give you an insightful perspective of where you spend your time and energy. This knowledge will be helpful in evaluating why you focus your attention there. See how your wheel turns, and observe what areas may be causing you to "clunk"

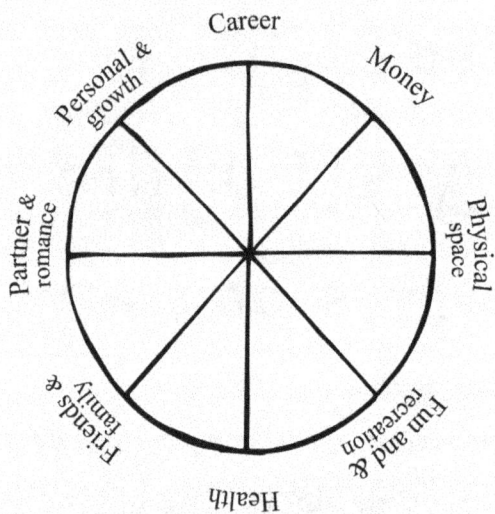

Career

Money

Physical space

Fun and & recreation

Health

Friends & family

Partner & romance

Personal & growth

Bedtime story for your inner child - How big is your rock?

One day, an expert in time management was speaking to a group of business students and, to drive home a point, used an illustration those students will never forget. As he stood in front of the group of high-powered over-achievers, he said, "Okay, time for a quiz" and he pulled out a one-gallon, wide-mouth Mason jar and set it on the table in front of him. He also produced about a dozen fist-sized rocks and carefully placed them, one at a time, into the jar.

When the jar was filled to the top and no more rocks would fit inside, he asked, "Is this jar full?" Everyone in the class yelled, "Yes." The time management expert replied, "Really?" He reached under the table and pulled out a bucket of gravel. He dumped some gravel in and shook the jar, causing pieces of gravel to work themselves down into the spaces between the big rocks. He then asked the group once more, "Is the jar full?" By this time the class was on to him. "Probably not," one of them answered. "Good!" he replied.

He reached under the table and brought out a bucket of sand. He started dumping the sand in the jar and it went into all of the spaces left between the rocks and the gravel. Once more he asked the question, "Is this jar full?" "No!" the class shouted. Once again he said, "Good." Then he grabbed a pitcher of water and began to pour it in until the jar was filled to the brim.

Then he looked at the class and asked, "What is the point of this illustration?" One eager beaver raised his hand and said, "The point is, no matter how full your schedule is, if you try really hard you can always fit some more things in it!"

"No," the speaker replied, "that's not the point. The truth this illustration teaches us is, "If you don't put the big rocks in first, you'll never get them in at all. What are the 'big rocks' in your life? Time with loved ones, your faith, your education, your dreams, a worthy cause, teaching or mentoring others. Remember to put these BIG ROCKS in first or they won't fit."

So, tonight, or in the morning, when you are reflecting on this short story, ask yourself this question, "What are the 'big rocks' in my life?" Then, put those in your jar first.

CHAPTER 4 –

THIS IS WHERE IT GETS REALLY INTERESTING!

You are pregnant

However you conceived, sitting with the news of your pregnancy is an incredible time. It's like a part of you has travelled to the edge of the universe and picked up a hitch-hiker. You know they are there, though it feels so unreal, yet at other times it feels like they have completely taken over your life and you haven't even meet them yet! Whatever your belief system is, you have a growing bud of life in you. A life that is at this stage completely dependent on you and your actions. You will be setting down the fine print, through your hormones and information substance to grow and nurture your baby. You are creating the hard drive for your baby's life. This is a seed that needs to be placed in a nurturing, relaxed and loving environment to maximize their full potential.

Stress, appraisal and coping

The brain is composed of two parts, the left and right hemisphere that interconnect through a massive network of nerves called the corpus callosum. Life can often feel like the mystical image of

Plato's Phaedrus metaphor, which likens the human psyche to a chariot being drawn by two horses. One white, one black. Both horses pulling in different directions and weakly controlled by a charioteer

The horses depict the neocortex of the human brain, which contains the parts of the brain that deal with conscious thought control, such as reasoning, understanding and decision-making. It also coordinates all voluntary muscle movement.

The unconscious mind or shadow is the charioteer, driving our lives. This is where most of the work gets done; it's the repository for automatic skills, like giving birth, and also the source of intuition and dreams through our emotional center, the engine of much information processing while we sleep. Fleeting perceptions register on the unconscious mind long before we may be aware of them, but they direct our actions. The unconscious mind is the source of hidden beliefs, fears and attitudes that interfere with everyday life and as we examine them we can choose how to meet with them.

The reptilian brain is the hard drive, responsible for our core and instinctive functioning, like self-preservation, reproduction and breathing. We use the reptilian brain to explore our environment, responding to danger with our "fight or flight" response.

This depicts how we might see the workings of conflicting values in our "pregnancy brain"

Illustration by Miah Fraser

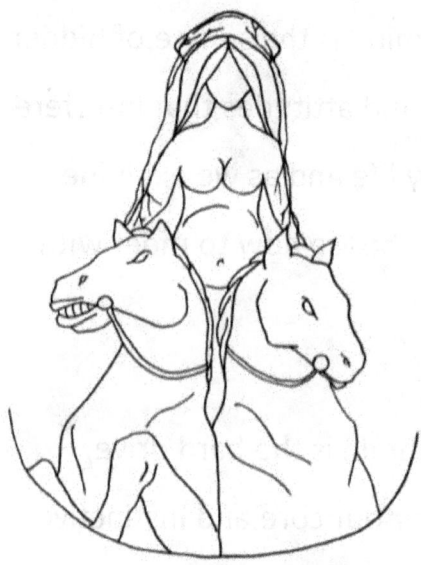

In normal life, we are able to coordinate the two horses, to travel fairly smoothly through the journey and create the life we want. In this way, our processes are congruent with each other, and we are able to create a life that keeps us happy. However, pregnancy is dependent on a complex range of events within the body, and if you experienced a traumatic birth as a baby, your body maybe sending out mixed messages about what is "normal" for it.

To fully understand why this applies to your pregnancy, we first need to look at a couple more things: the body's physiological response to stress, and our appraisal mechanisms, or how we perceive stress. This explains why the stories that are constructed around our identities are so important to us. How can we safely change our response to stressful triggers to manage it in terms of our pregnancy?

Myth # 4 - Stress is the same for everybody, and only major symptoms of stress require your attention

How you appraise the presence of stress in your life may have a direct influence on the outcome of you pregnancy and your relationship with your baby. Stress is not intrinsic to a situation but arises from a person's appraisal of events as being too dangerous to manage and leaves you feeling as though your resources have been taxed. Appraisal is extremely individual and is influenced through a complex pathway of personal meanings, the context of events, and repetition compulsion association verses condition response.

Your response to stressful events can be divided into two types of reactions, termed "appraisal." Primary appraisal involves assessing the environmental situation with regard to your safety and evaluating three options. The first response to the stressors is considered irrelevant because you perceive there is no real threat. The event is not stressful and it holds no impact for you. Michelle describes her wedding, for example, as a "lovely day, a great time."

Case study

Rosie – And did you plan it yourself?

Michelle –*"Yep, yes it was good, it was fun, and I don't know or understand anyone that gets stressed or anything*

about planning a wedding"

Rosie – What was the thing you enjoyed

most about it?

Michelle –*"Just really the anticipation of*

just having everyone there and having a

good time and we all just sort of partied

together more than anything."

Many people rate getting married as

highly stressful, yet Michelle appeared to

be taking it all in her stride. She has

strongly developed skills that allow her to

manage her reactions through conscious

process.

The second response that you can have to the stressful stimuli is considered benign or even positive for you. Michelle describes house hunting as a pleasure.

Rosie –Anything else that was going on in your life prior to you becoming pregnant?

Michelle – *"Um not really. We were looking for a house, but we were looking at houses for so long and it wasn't overly urgent either so OK that's just what you do on a Saturday um and yeah nothing really else like I just sort of work and friends and my husband and um"*

The third response is that the event is recognized as stressful, such as when Michelle gave birth to her twenty-four week old son. The event stimulated a secondary appraisal mechanism in which Michelle evaluated whether they can eliminate the source of stress and how they would manage it

Rosie – So being busy is one of your coping mechanisms?

Michelle – *"Yes, yes definately and also um yeah, like I never really, like I never got too emotional like I made a rule pretty early on that nobody cries next to our baby's bed, like, and ...."*

Rosie – Why did you decide that?

Michelle – *"I thought so OK he needs positive vibes so I just like it just doesn't help anyone, it doesn't help me, if I've been crying, it doesn't help the nurses who have things to do and I had one, I think I had one bit of a breakdown in the labour ward, I just thought nobody was there and I had to express and it didn't work out at all. I didn't have colostrums and the midwives were busy coming and then, I think then on top of that, you know, how these random people just walk in and want to talk to you about something and I just lost it big time but that was the only time I can really, really remember sort of being...(out of control)"*

Being aware of effective coping mechanisms allows you to diminishes & control the stress, in most cases of acute stress. However, stress will be experienced as traumatic if the appraisal is deemed as threatening, or the person perceives they do not have sufficient coping strategies. This manifests in a very complex way within the body. Michelle gives us an insight into how she managed the birth of her son.

Rosie – How did you manage that?

Michelle – *"well I didn't have a choice, it's really - that's the bottom line and I think everyone has some sort of coping mechanisms and I think I have quite good ones and you just switch into this, like I switch into this - I sort of, I tend to shut out emotions a lot. I tend to not be very emotional. A lot of people just expected me to break down crying but I didn't have the energy for it so I somehow thought, "I've somehow got to get through this" and I just blanked out a lot. Like my husband, he cried a lot. He was a lot more emotionally upset than I*

was but that probably helped, like I had
all the expressing of milk and that sort of
things around me to worry about"

Stress and fear imposes a profoundly
negative effect on your body. Although it
is biologically important to notice and
respond to the warning signs produced by
stress and fear, such fear is seldom good
for us. Paradoxically, many times it only
gets in the way. Instead of saving our
lives, as we are informed it does in the
fight & flight response fear often keeps us
from living our lives to the full.

If we have failed in the past, we respond
to fear on the basis of an unconscious

faulty conclusion about our capacity to manage our future. Our typical inherently self-defeating responses to fear keep us from tapping into our full potential.

The process of evaluating the demands made of you occurs not only at the onset of the event, but during the course of the event as well. It is this interaction over time that constitutes your appraisal process and modulates the degree of stress experienced.

A chain of events

When an individual appraises stressors as demanding or threatening, two principal physiological reactions occur. One involves the autonomic system, where adrenaline and noradrenaline, known as catecholamines, are released into your body.

The other involves the hypothalamic-pituitary-adrenal (HPA) axis, whereby the release of corticotrophin releasing hormones (CHR) and adrenocorticotropic hormone (ACTH), and cortisol, which is the predominate agent that cause of that feeling of fear in your body. Both reactions occur in the brain as a response from our nervous system, which feeds back from our senses. What we see, hear, smell, touch, think and feel affects us.

Activation of these responses in your body alters your behavior, such as eating and sleeping. You may feel more anxious or depressed as your sense of well-being is diminished. You may even begin to experience hyperarousal or hypervigilance of the senses. You will notice that your sleep will become disturbed due to your pregnancy. It's not just your aching bones, swollen feet and pressing bladder that cause this. They are simply the symptoms of the experience.

Your body and your baby are changing in preparation for the biggest event in your life so far, yet long-term activation of these two systems causes fatigue, with a resulting effect of your body being unable to respond properly. One key factor in countering this is to break the response and learn to relax, giving other good hormones available in your body a chance to do their work. If you try, it happens easily in pregnancy – that's one of the fun parts of the process. Enjoy it while you can!

Labour

The onset of labour results from an intricate interplay between the maternal, fetal, placental endocrine systems and information substances systems. This will happen inside you, without your conscious control. It involves complex positive and negative feedback systems, in cellular receptor sites, and dynamic chemical messenger systems. A cascade of events culminates in eventual maturation of the baby and the mother's uterine tissue, thereby stimulating birth to occur.

The placenta releases corticotrophin-releasing hormone (CRH) in increasing amounts throughout the pregnancy. This plays an important role in the time of the birth, as it is believed to be the process that matures the baby's organs for an independent life. An alteration in this process can have implications for both you and your baby. Research has suggested that high levels of CRH in early to mid-pregnancy can be indicative of a preterm birth process. High levels of CRH cause the baby's organs to mature for independent life quickly. As the baby's tissues respond, they send out chemical messages, along with the CHR released from both mother and placenta, to the uterine muscles, to start contractions and soften the cervix to open for birth.

Higher production of CHR produced in the mother through her stress response, combines with and stimulates the placenta to produce more CHR. These combined high levels of CHR mature the baby's organs and uterine wall for an early birth. Further studies continue to explore the concept that chronic stress in pregnant women can be a major cause in idiopathic preterm birth.

Myth # 4 busted!

OK, so why is this important information? Having the facts about something allows you to rationalize your feelings and body responses. Understanding what is happening and why. This allows you to stay in control. Let's look at what this may feel like for a normal vaginal birth.

First of all you have to get to term. Your baby has finished developing and the last month or two, it's just hanging around getting fat and maturing. This is good for the baby, but by this time most women start to feel like they've had enough.

There are normally a variety of pains and discomforts in the body, experienced through the changes of pregnancy, which if added up supersede any pain of birth. Nature is preparing us to have confidence in our ability to work through these discomforts. One step at a time.

Journal activity

Make notes in your journal of all the various aches and pains during your pregnancy. Score them on a subjective scale (SUDS) from 0 – 10; 0 is no pain or discomfort at all, while 10, which is unbearable, and requires medical assistance. Please take the time to do this. Our mind has a great way of playing tricks on us and I have found that if you document something in the moment, it will give you a real tool to do subjective work with as you approach your birth. It is completely normal to wonder throughout the length of your pregnancy "how the hell

am I going to get this out of my body?"
Many of us can't bear to think about it,
finding the very idea overwhelming! You are
not alone. But you can think about what is
happening right now. Write down your pain
scores. Write down how you managed, and
take note – you survived it.

Changing State of Being

As I approached full term, and birth became imminent, I like many other women experienced a change in my state of being. I went from being fearful of my birth process to not caring! I didn't care how the baby came out – I just wanted it out. It's as though the unconscious, chemical part of my system simply changed how I felt about it. I, as in my conscious brain, moved aside to let the process take over and it remains to this day the most amazing process in my life.

Stress is complex but universal, something we all experience. Internal and external triggers can stimulate it and we develop coping skills to protect ourselves from it. Protective factors include our behaviour and lifestyle factors. External protective factors, which are considered part of the environment, can be seen as family, social support networks and the unexpected events that shape the women's journey. Internal protective factors are our beliefs and values.

Sliding scale of responses

Repetition compulsion is an accepted psychological phenomenon in which you repeat a traumatic or painful event and its circumstances over and over again in your life. This includes reenacting the event or putting your self in situations where the event is likely to happen again. This "re-living" can also take the form of night mares in which memories and feelings of what happened are repeated. It is driven by the mid brain and not consciously controlled. This part of your brain doesn't really respond to spoken command or thought, but can be communicated best through image to illicit a feeling and response.

Freud describes the pattern whereby people endlessly repeat patterns of behavior which were difficult or distressing in earlier life as though they were trying to resolve, or problem solve them. As we are creatures of meaning and reasoning, we repeatedly try to solve our deepest traumas.

The term conditioned reflex was first used by Pavlov to describe a reflex which is acquired, rather than inborn. It is what we learn through repetition compulsion actions. It is also peculiar to the individual rather than the whole species. It differs from an unconditional response, such as a newborn's sucking response because it has been learnt or developed in life.

Often, decision-making can become difficult because we are bombarded with information, both factual and fictitious. This information is processed inside ourselves through our hopes, dreams and ambitions, and the world outside ourselves, where we are assessed, judged and restrained from being ourselves.

Yet one opinion of reality is that we are not fixed identities that view life and its events from a beneficial vantage point, but rather we slide through a spectrum of awarenesses. Like a pendulum swings from side to side or around and around. This sliding scale of responses is a more accepting way to manage events. If we can get our conscious minds on board with what's happening in our subconscious, and not vice-versa, we will be heading for a much smoother journey into motherhood.

Case study

Michelle describes how strength in one situation can be a weakness in another, but relationships can serve as external protective factors, and she was still able to manage the stressful event by letting go. Michelle describes how her sister-in-law, Katie, visited her on the day she went into labor. Katie is an experienced midwife and also knows how Michelle manages events. Michelle's coping strategy was to minimalize or downplay her symptoms for fear of being labeled a hypochondriac.

Michelle – *"My sister in law was there which was good. This was really a coincidence because she just popped in really, on the way home from work. She was actually the one who said –because that is my way. I'm always the one to say "I'm alright, I'm alright"– and she was like "well you're not alright! You're like going into labour– you've got to tell them that", and she was on my back about that. I think she was quite good because then actually a doctor came and realized, OK, this woman is dilated. We think it's going to be going to happen, were as I would have just kept, just kept lying there alright, in my "I'm OK" kind of thing."*

Rosie – Because you were so, trying to hold it in?

Michelle –*"Yes and also, I don't know! That's just how I am. It's a bit, as well like - not a….. that's why it's really weird for me to be here at all, because I'm not like a hypochondriac whiner but like, I'm here all the time so... because you just don't know, what, like how to react! Like I always envisaged I'd be really happy or elated, excited, but there was just nothing I just sort of felt empty, deflated and sort of quite scared as to what's going on, so yes."*

The Summary

Appraisal is a personal examination of the effect of exposure of the individual self to life stressors.

Meaning is gained through assessing psychological appraisal and emotional response in regards to life events and their context, which is assessment of the environmental demands and daily events or chronic stressors.

Resiliency, resourcefulness and coping strategies are factors or tools that can be adapted and sufficient to manage the stress load, depending on the amount of psychosocial support you feel you are receiving.

Major life stressors can have a positive as well as negative effect on psychological well-being as the event unfolds. Cognitive adaption and coping strategies illustrate how appraisals can help you restore a sense of control and find meaning in the event. Reappraising a threatening experience as beneficial or gainful brings meaning to the event.

Meaning is attributed on the basis of perceived severity and implications of the personal values and expectations. There are external factors in your life like money, how people project back onto you, your sense of self-esteem and what you expect to happen or what your assumptions of the event are. Your variables or internal factors will form parts of your "pregnant woman's identity", which are bought into the appraisal of new events that occur through the experience of being pregnant.

Quick Quiz # 6 – What's your "pea" telling you?

Below is a list of the most stressful major life events one is likely to experience.

Plot out what you have experienced. Observe your recovery time and access your acute and chronic life event episodes. Add your own events to the list and observe what helped you most through these events and record what you believe you learnt from them.

- Death of a spouse
- Jail sentence
- Death of immediate family member
- Immediate family member commits suicide
- Getting into debt beyond means of repayment
- Period of homelessness
- Seriously illness
- Moving house
- Unemployment
- Marriage
- Divorce.
- Break up of family
- Moving countries.
- Injury or illness.
- Unhappy or bullied at work.
- Fired from your work

Journal activity

Design and label a drawing or symbol for
your journal that identifies your events so
far. List your internal and external
protective factors. Remember, this is not a
competition, but a self-awareness exercise
to help you and your baby. Immerse
yourself in it for an evening or so and see
what you come up with. Remember, this is
not a fixed set list, and it will change with
time as you and your baby experience more
life together.

Bedtime story- Hans Christian Andersen The Princess and the Pea

Once upon a time there was a prince who wanted to marry a princess, but she would have to be a real princess. He travelled all over the world to find one, but nowhere could he get what he wanted. There were princesses enough, but it was difficult to find out whether they were real ones. There was always something about them that was not as it should be. So he came home again and was sad, for he would have liked very much to have a real princess.

One evening a terrible storm came on; there was thunder and lightning, and the rain poured down in torrents. Suddenly a knocking was heard at the city gate, and the old king went to open it.

It was a princess standing out there in front of the gate. But, good gracious! What a sight the rain and the wind had made her. The water ran down from her hair and clothes; it ran down into the toes of her shoes and out again at the heels. And yet she said that she was a real princess.

Well, we'll soon find that out, thought the old queen. But she said nothing, went into the bedroom, took all the bedding off the bedstead, and laid a pea on the bottom; then she took twenty mattresses and laid them on the pea, and then twenty eider-down beds on top of the mattresses.

On this the princess had to lie all night. In the morning she was asked how she had slept.

"Oh, very badly!" said she. "I have scarcely closed my eyes all night. Heaven only knows what was in the bed, but I was lying on something hard, so that I am black and blue all over my body. It's horrible!"

Now they knew that she was a real princess because she had felt the pea right through the twenty mattresses and the twenty eider-down beds.

Nobody but a real princess could be as sensitive as that.
So the prince took her for his wife, for now he knew that he had a real princess; and the pea was put in the museum, where it may still be seen, if no one has stolen it.

There, that is a true story.

(Adapted from the story by Hans Christian Andersen.)

CHAPTER FIVE –

PLOTTING THE JOURNEY

Prevention is better than cure

As mentioned in Chapter Two, identity is constructed through relationship, so getting to know your pregnancy is important. To do this you need to find some time to take a snapshot of where you are now. Let's map out what else is going on in your life.

In Quick quiz # 4 we were able to name the roles that we already play in our life. Print out the circles from the sheet below. Place yourself at the center, just say ME, and then in order of your priority label the consecutive circles from the center outwards with your other identities.

You may find that you begin to have conflict between internal drives and external drives. For instance, being a "student" and spending time on my studies is in conflict with my need to work and make money. I spend more time "working", than I do in formal study, but my passion is to continue learning. So although I spend 40 hours a week on my work, and only eight hours on my study projects I would place them both at the core of my center.

Having a neat, beautiful home is important to me, and I have developed great time management skills through my years, but having a perfect home has to be placed to the outer edges of my circle. It's just not that important to me in the scale of things, to live a picture perfect life. I prefer to have the experience of constantly developing myself over having an impeccably tidy home. However I know lots of women whom I love and respect but whose values are different to mine.

It is important to them to have everything in place. They are not prepared to drop that standard in their life and accommodate the needs of their family around that. There really is no right or wrong way; it comes down to your preferences, your management and what's available to you.

Quick quiz # 7 – Prioritising my identities

Taking your "Labels" from Chapter Two, give yourself time to think about your life and all the roles you play. Place them on the circles in order of meaning for you, with the most valuable at the center. You can change their position whenever you want. Nothing is permanent, feelings change. The circles will help you gain clarity in your changing roles and identity

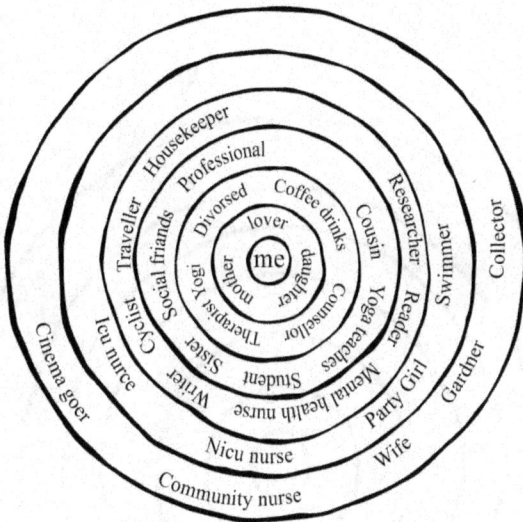

Print and enter your
own identities
according to your
values

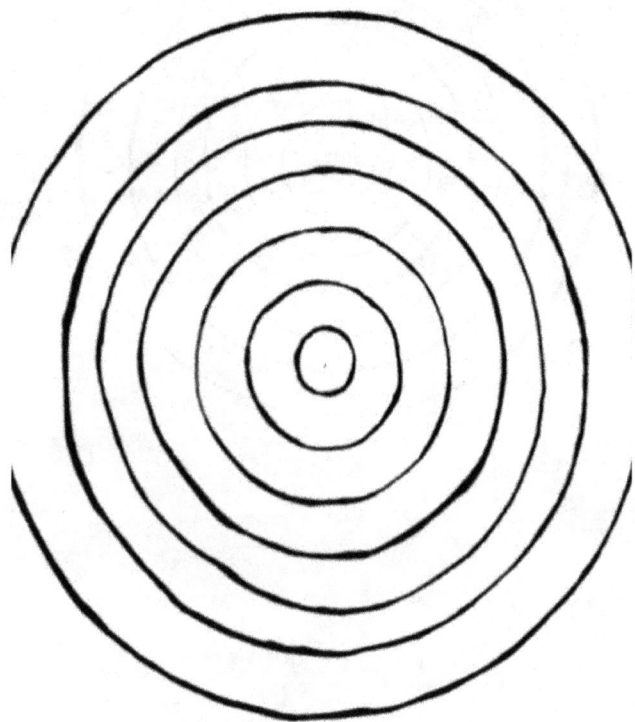

Myth # 5 – A woman always glows when she is pregnant!

For some women, pregnancy is a state of grace during which they are fully supported, loved and appreciated, have minimal discomforts in their pregnancy, endure no outside pressures – they seem to blossom! If this is you, please recognize that you are among the lucky ones and you are blessed. This is not the experience many women have as they go through the process of growing another human being in their bodies. The experience of being pregnant, if they get the chance to have it, is often so different from what they expected or imagined.

Pregnancy may be stressful, with a combination of events creating this for the women; antenatal illness, change in body image, change in relationship with your partner, change in identity, unplanned delivery, fear for survival of the baby, aches and pains, lack of sleep, and financial pressures may lead to adapted physical and psychological responses. This can be hard to deal with. People expect you to be happy. However, knowing that there is a flip side to pregnancy can be helpful. Not ignoring your reactions is imperative to being able to manage them.

Case study

Zoe is a 32-year-old professional who works in the health industry. She is happily married, but lives away from her family, who live in South Africa.
Zoe describes her initial reactions to her expectations about being pregnant.

Zoe – "Well you know, your initial expectations are like, when you're younger, you know. It's lovely to see a pregnant lady and then the next time you see her, there she is, walking down

the street with this beautiful baby and
stuff like - I never really felt that, I never
felt nice in my pregnancy at all" .

Zoe was a student of mine who had
desperately wanted a baby. Now, she
loves her baby and is a wonderful
mother. But she had experienced
multiple miscarriages in the past in the
first trimester of her pregnancy. She
describes her expectations of pregnancy.

Zoe - *"Yeah, well I didn't have any real*
expectations. I just I expected that I
would enjoy it a lot more but I was a bit
grossed out by the whole kicking thing,
[and] when he rolled, I lost my whole

stomach, like my whole stomach was actually deformed."

Not everyone finds pregnancy as they expected it to be. She describes her reaction to some of the events in her pregnancy.

Zoe –*"I was quite upset that I was grossed out by it so much. Yeah, I just I thought I'd enjoy it more. I thought I'd be this beautiful glowing thing you know. A happiness person but I wasn't. I was in my final year of uni doing my degree and you know I was cutting it very fine in terms of exams and things; he was due on my very last day of my last exam so it wasn't really a stress free period."*

What is interesting here is that Zoe's baby listened to her, but unfortunately she had to be induced as she went well over her due date. Her baby had begun to over mature inside her and as a result its system had started to 'poo' inside her. This is medically termed passing meconium into the amniotic fluid, which then moves into the baby's lungs through the birth process, and can result in a life-threatening lung infection for the baby.

We draw our assumptions or expectations of the world from past and present events. Past experiences inform us, through our reflecting process and by how we act out in our lives. We reconnect to old memories, re-live conversations and events in our heads when we have the time to sit quietly with ourselves, we experience them through our dreams, and display them in action as we speak, through our unconscious words and actions as we move through our day.

Hopes, dreams and aspirations are our projections into the future. Through our hopes, dreams and goal setting process, we build an image of what we want our lives to look like. Disappointment occurs when these two things don't connect properly into the present moment. And by sitting with the present, through the facts of the moment we can tell what is real in our worlds.

We draw on outside events, things that happened to us, but also to people we know, and stories that we have heard. We draw on our responses to those events, whether we have judged them to be positive or negative, good or bad. Those binary labels that lead us to thinking in fixed outcomes. Our emotional brain can't actually distinguish between fact and fiction. That is the process of our conscious brain. Yet our emotional brain is what drives the chariot in our lives.

I can't really think of any other area in a busy woman's life were we have so much freedom of choice, yet take so little action to make the most of these opportunities for ourselves, our babies and our families.

Journal activity

Where have you formed

your view of pregnancy?

How does it look for you?

Quick Quiz # 8– Is this helpful or unhelpful?

Make a list of the people, places and events that have informed you about pregnancy. Once you start writing you will be surprised by how much information you have already acquired. Don't analyze the process. Just empty your mind onto a page, in the fashion that you use to brainstorm, or mind map.

Think of stories and events that leave you feeling secure about what you know, and have already achieved. Qualities that stand out for you as important in understanding who you are and why you want your baby. No one can tell you what should be on your list. Knowing yourself and your values will help prepare you for motherhood. You have a lot to organize, in the next few months. It is fun to understand what drives your motives so that you can draw on them if the pressure increases and things get challenging in the future.

Quick Quiz # 9 – What is your preference?

Make three columns with the headings "clinical", "superficial" and "meaningful". Now list the information from your brain storming session into the right columns for you. How is your information weighted? What preferences does it highlight for you?

Let's start to change how we see
the situation by changing what we
ask. It is about recognition, not
judgment. Each time we arrive at an
appraisal, rather than going to the
dichotomy of good or bad, try asking,
"is this helpful or unhelpful"? Create
a SUDS scale of 0- 10, and mark
down where you place the
experience in terms of its influence
on you. Then explore what parts of
it are helpful and what parts are
unhelpful. There are very few events
in life that are absolutely one or the
other.

Consider what was significant about this exercise for you?

What did you learn or what was reinforced about yourself?

What patterns do you see forming?

What can you take from this activities to use in your life?

Case study

Your pregnancy will be even more stimulating for you as you begin to realize the importance of the implications of your own reflection. Creating a relationship with your pregnancy by actively engaging with the journey. There are those who believe as I do that if deep, meaningful, long-lasting learning is left to chance a strategic and integrated part of the pregnancy process will be missed. Pregnancy is, after all, all about growth.

Michelle was able to give an insightful response when she was asked how she had formed her views of pregnancy.

Michelle – *"probably friends who had children, quite a few, two of my really good friends had children a year and a half before me and I think mainly through them. At home my cousins are really basically our age, like my sisters and mine, I mean. Nobody in my family was ever pregnant because my sister, I was two when my sister was born so I have no recollection of that so yeah I would say I would say friends. Just people I would consider being similar to myself."*

Michelle was able to identify the women in her life who were most influential. Yet she missed making the connection to her own birth story, and the details of her mother's pregnancy with her. It was only with prompting that Michelle was able to disclosed vital information that may have made a difference to how her first pregnancy was managed, yet she still didn't connect the dots and reflect upon the meaningful information available to her.

Rosie – Do you remember any stories around your mum's pregnancy?

Michelle – *"She was very sick, I think, right to the end. I know she had to sort of get off the train at least once to vomit and it was on the way to work. I know she had her cervix soften so she had to have a circlet put in and I think she got it put in quite early. I just knew that after birth, I think both of us were taken straight away because I was very jaundiced so they just, I think they just put us into an ambulance and drove to the children's hospital and that was a bit traumatic for my mum."*

Rosie – So both her babies were taken away?

Michelle – *"Yeah and I often think back then like in the seventies they didn't think so much about the mother. They just sort of said "OK make sure the baby's alright –"let's go."*

Myth # 5
busted

The medical world provides us with clinical information. They are trained in the latest obstetric practices and have invested many years of their lives to be able to assist you and trusting your practitioner is an essential component to feeling safe in your birth. They will ask you lots of questions and your ability to give an informed answer is essential to the quality of care you receive. As you are going through a unique and new process for yourself how do you know what the right question for you to ask are? How do you know what you don't know?

Critical reflection is an important part of any learning process. Without reflection, your pregnancy can become only a distracting activity — like viewing a reality TV show — which was never meant to have meaning, merely to occupy your time.

Reflection is not meditation, rather it is *mediation* — an active, dialectical exercise that requires as much intellectual work from analysis to evaluation. But in reflection, all the learned material can be gathered about, sorted and resorted, and searched through for greater understanding and inspiration, thus allowing all parts of our brain to take in this information,

recognize what it knows and make

meaning of the process.

Creating support for yourself and your

baby is not just about financial security,

having the latest look, or going to the

right places and rushing around. Support

can be found in how we view ourselves,

how we talk to ourselves and how much

time we give ourselves, through

befriending our changing body.

Bedtime story – Friends are a gift by Kerry Armstrong

A wonderful part of life. An unexpected surprise.

A friend is a companion, someone you can talk to, who'll listen and laugh with you.

A true friend won't let you down, but will help you through the rough bits, and carry you through the times when you think you can't go on.

A friend will back you up, won't run you down or talk behind your back.A friend will love you and your loved ones, but would never take advantage of you or betray you.

A friend will keep your inner most secrets safe.

Value your beliefs and dreams.
Uphold and honor your morals.
Understand you.
And let you be yourself.

And then there are the people who say
they are your friends, but:
Undermine you.
Deplete you.
Let you down.
Try to change you.
Take away your faith in yourself.

In times like these, I help myself.

CHAPTER SIX –

THERE ARE TWO SIDES TO EVERY STORY

All roads lead to Rome

If you're worried about giving birth, you're not alone. After coaching women on this subject for nearly 20 years, I can assure you that you are keeping very good company and I would be surprised if someone arrived in my class and wasn't scared. We are hard wired to have at least some fear during this momentous event, whether by a natural or any other form of delivery. All roads lead to Rome in this instance. You are giving birth.

There is no other identity shift that is as totalizing as this process. We are all hard wired to experience this deep within our brain, but we experience a massive conflict between our urge to procreate and our own self-preservation drive. The chemicals that are released within our busy bodies gear us up for the event anyway. We have no conscious control over the matter. We have to let go and trust our deepest self.

Yet many women in our culture are completely unprepared for this. They draw their ideas of birth from contemporary culture, through movies, TV and books, as more and more of our population becomes transient and we lose our ties with our extended families and our cultural understanding of what birth is for us. We lose the connection to the reality of the situation. We are informed by images of soap stars and super models.

All of the women in my study group and most of my students in my classes live away from their family of origin. As strong young women, many of us moved away from home to travel and experience life. We meet partners from abroad, or different parts of Australia and settled in a new area. But in doing so, we have lost a close connection to their extended family. Some women just grew up without experiencing another baby in the household, as their parents, or grandparents had made these moves for them.

How we have formed our expectations of pregnancy, birth and motherhood will be impacted by and reflect the current cultural values in our communities. We are privileged to live in First World countries with an amazing health system that keeps us safe. However, we have to do our part. I invite you now to consider how you formed your opinion of pregnancy. What events, and which people influenced you, and explore how this may indicate how well we are able to transition to the role of mother.

Myth # 6 - The fruit doesn't fall too far from the tree!

Contemporary TV, media and the movie industry show a variety of images - real and fantasy - which portray the birthing women lying on her back, with her legs in stirrups. Pain relief is provided through an epidural as the baby is pulled from her body with forceps, or the women are rushed off to theatres for an emergency caesarean. These are actually the realities of my first experiences of birth when I was a student nurse. They are clinical.

The medical establishment and society wants a safer birth process for both mother and baby, which leads to a higher rate of intervention with births.

I invite you now to form the link between your own safe arrival onto the planet as a baby and your adult self. This may be a big ask initially for such a simple concept. But we are all more than survivors; we are winners, because despite difficult situations we come from a long line of survivors. All of our ancestors, all of our genetic identity has developed because they made it to adulthood, despite the adversity your relatives may have experienced, you are here now, with their knowledge imprinted in your genes to get you through.

The majority of my clients are able to take important information about their arrival into the world and learn from it. I myself missed the connection with my mother's birth story and around my own arrival into the world and the journey of my daughter. Our own innate knowledge can sometime be minimalized, and had I known then what I know now, I would have managed my first pregnancy differently.

I was born through a caesarean section in 1963. My mother underwent a general anaesthetic because she felt too tired to face another birth. She had three previous live births and one miscarriage. My sister had recently died in a cot death. My mother was fragile and exhausted. She was offered a caesarean section, but back then anaesthetics where not so refined and I needed resuscitation upon delivery. I was the first in my family to be born this way, yet never reflected on this until much later in my life.

The story of the birth of my children

At the time, I had just set up my first yoga school. I had owned it for three years and things were going well. I'd almost reached a place where I believed I wasn't going to conceive. After seven years in relationship without a conception, my thoughts were on enjoying my life. I had just married and spent about three months in India studying yoga with my gurus. I travelled a bit but most of my time was spent in practice, visiting ancient holy cities, and learning from my teachers and fellow yogis on the same path.

When I returned to Sydney, I conceived Kimberley. This was a busy time. I was still in conflict between the values of Eastern, Western and Celtic traditions and was learning a lot from other people. I had a very busy lifestyle. I was over active for Kimberley's pregnancy, although I rested when I could, I didn't want to let go of my cycling fitness, swimming in the surf and teaching twelve classes of yoga a week as well as running the business. I wanted our home to be ready for our baby. We needed to renovate and decorate and my nesting instincts kicked in strongly. I was lucky enough to do a week-long mediation with the Dalai Lama, where he blessed my belly. This was a beautiful occasion.

But by 32 weeks, Kimberley hadn't turned head down, into the best birth position. A Chinese medical practitioner informed me that this was an indication that my baby was trying to help me. To reassure me by taking her conscious part, her brain, towards my heart.

I was a trained intensive care nurse, and I had taught prenatal yoga for a number of years. I was desperate to have a natural birth. In my heart, mind and body I was ready to give birth. By 38 weeks Kimberley still hadn't turned and I had to make a decision. I was still feeling really confident that I could birth a breech baby with the right assistance. I was under the care of a senior obstetrician who had good skills for such deliveries and was booked into a birthing center that supported such births.

As I was walking to my final doctor's appointment, I met a young women who was as pregnant as me. We fell into conversation. She also owned a small business and said that this was her second baby. I was feeling tired, fat and busy. How did she do all I did and look after a toddler as well. I was impressed.

We enjoyed a meaningful, candid conversation in which we were able to connect and chat at length about these issues. She shared with me the story of her first labor. Her baby had been just like the one I was carrying at that time, breech and not wanting to turn. She had followed her heart and went with a natural delivery, and explained how her baby had died during the birth. It was no one's fault, but part of her process.

Instantly my decision making process had changed. This wasn't about me wanting to do a natural birth. It was about me making responsible decisions as a mother. It was about my baby and her safety. I went to the doctor's and booked a planned caesarean section.

Kimberley Rose - The clinical

Kimberley Rose was born via a planned caesarean section on 18 November, 1996. She was a breech presentation and I never tried to turn her as I thought her to be headstrong and independent. I was in hospital for three days with a catheter and experienced a CSF leak from the insertion of my epidural. Rather than going back to theatre for a "spinal patch," I healed my spine through yoga, NET, homeopathic and chiropractic techniques.

The morning I was going for my appointment to make a decision on my delivery style, I met a woman who had lost her baby through a natural breech delivery.

I am so glad I never risked my baby - she is beautiful! She is also the model for the peaceful, reflective baby in the book cover.

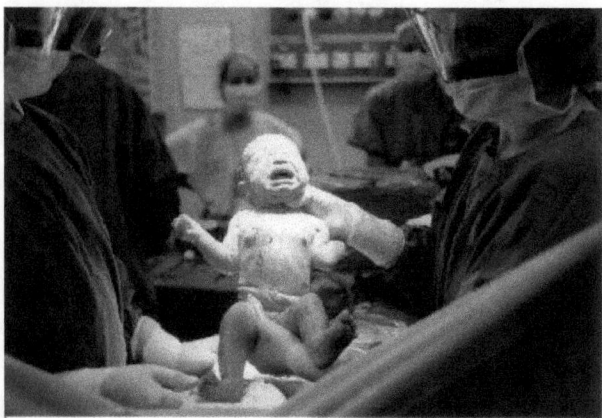

Kimberley at birth

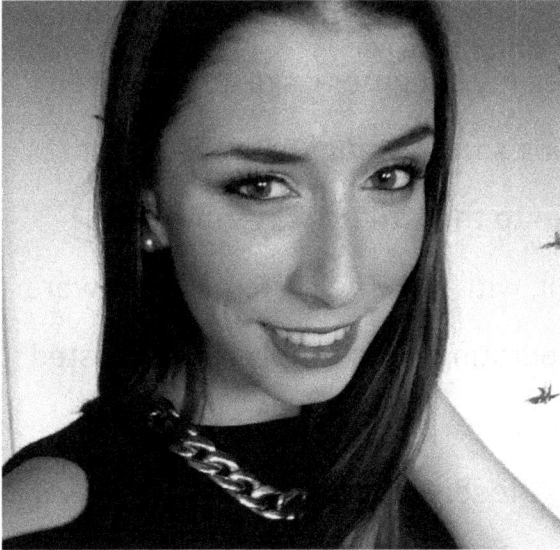

Kimberley at 17

Continuing my story

With Kimberley born, I was still running my business and planning a six month trip back to the UK. My husband had some locum work in Oxford, conveniently located for us to visit family and friends and show off our beautiful daughter.

I quickly met some new friends, who had babies my daughter's age, and enjoyed sharing social outings with them. But I began to think there was something wrong with me. Their energy levels were recuperating but I simply felt exhausted all the time. I was passionate about breast-feeding Kimberley and was upset that she was a "fussy" eater, yet spent a lot of time persevering. Things were spiralling downhill fast, with so much going on in my life. I thought I should feel great – but I didn't.

I was just about to make an appointment with the health visitor, believing myself to be suffering from depression, when I suddenly had an epiphany that I was pregnant. I couldn't even entertain the thought. How could I be pregnant again? Kimberley was only five months old, I was breastfeeding, and for god's sake I couldn't even remember having sex!

But the feeling persisted. The next day I picked up a home pregnancy test with the shopping, feeling ridiculous with myself for doing so. As I walked into the house my husband was on the phone with an old college friend when I overheard him say "Oh really, your wife is pregnant again? But I thought you already had a toddler?" It felt surreal as I went into the bathroom and performed the test. I did one, then another, just to make sure. My husband came upstairs to see what was taking so long and I showed him the tests. I waited for him to show a reaction before I could register a thought. He was delighted, with a snap of his fingers, the smile on his face and the twinkle in his eye I allowed myself to embrace the idea that I was going to have another baby. But I already realized I had to take a different approach to this baby.

Things were still busy. We had a three-week trip planned for Portugal when all I wanted to do was nest. I felt sad and guilty for taking Kimberley off the breast at only six month old. But she transitioned well to solids and a bottle all at the same time. Robert was already five months from conception and I had to say good-bye to my family in England and return to Australia to sell my beloved yoga center. I realized I couldn't do it all and made the decision to focus on my family.

Robert Angus – a natural

Robert Angus was born on 25 December 1997 just 13 months after Kimberley arrived in the world and just one week after she had started walking.

As you may notice Robert was born on Christmas Day, just like his dad, and joking aside, I swear he was an immaculate conception because I never planned to have two children so close together. However, after the initial shock, I accepted Roberts's arrival and changed some of my practices to accommodate him.

Mild contractions started in the morning as we opened presents. My waters broke at about 3pm and I was in hospital by 5pm. Robert was born two hours and fifteen minutes later, with a natural birth process: no gas, drugs or intervention. I

was home by 11pm that night. Roberts's

birth is the best thing I've ever done...

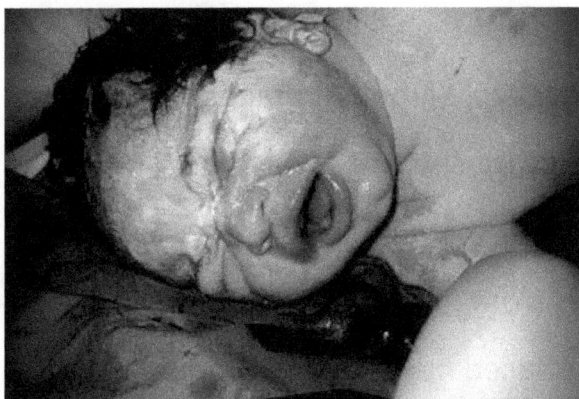

Robert at birth and Robert at 16

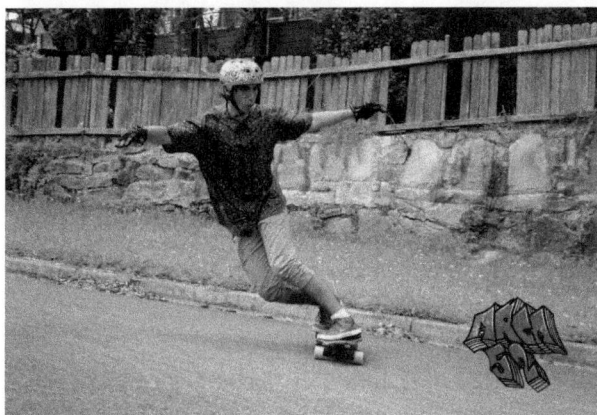

I only started reflecting on my own

journey into the world, and how this

influenced the birth of my daughter when I came across a process called Neuro Emotional Technique, or NET. This belongs to a group of practices called energy psychology. Whilst the chiropractor was healing my back and scars from the birth of Kimberley, he introduced me to this technique, which has influenced me greatly.

Neuro Emotional Technique –NET

I am an advanced certified NET practitioner. NET is a mind-body stress-reduction technique that uses a methodology of finding and removing neurological imbalances related to an unresolved mind-body component. NET is a tool that is used by practitioners of all disciplines to help improve behavioural and physical conditions. NET is a Mind-Body stress relief technique that has generated an incredible amount of excitement since 1988 and is very effective.

Journal Activity

Write down what you know of your own birth story. This is your original event and although you may not consciously make sense of the information, reflecting on it will help your subconscious process it.

Write a story, poem or letter to yourself describing the events in third person. Record it on your phone and play it back to yourself, or become really creative: draw, paint or design an image or picture of your story. Reflect on what comes out as a result.

When you are in a place of deep relaxation, run your mind through the events of your own birth.

Connect to your breath and relax. What emotions emerge? Just breathe them through. This has meaning for you at the deepest cellular level, can you reconnect with it? Be aware of the feelings as they come up but don't hold onto them. Let they go, let them drift away. Know that you have made this journey before and you survived. You are a survivor: trust yourself, trust your process and let go.

Without this clarity, your efforts to keep a balance between meeting your needs and coping with the pressures of your changing life are taking place in the dark. This can keep you from finding the peacefulness in your pregnancy. Try not to rush through your process.

Myth # 6 –
Myth confirmed

I was really surprised by the link between my own birth story and that of my daughter. My mother was pretty vague about it as I was her fourth child. I was also a breech presentation and she had me as an emergency caesarean section with a general anaesthetic. I will remember the scars on her belly forever.

It was only after speaking to many women about it that I realized there was a connection between how our mothers birthed and how we birth our babies. Yet the importance of this information seems lost to us all. Statistics support this theory: high intervention and pre term births are becoming more common because they are cyclic in nature and move from one generation to the next. Breaking the cycle requires a conscious choice. This needs to be worked with throughout the pregnancy and can take many shapes, forms or actions in its doing. There are no guarantees to the process. It's not what you do that matters, but the way that you do it. Develop awareness and accept the outcomes.

Bedtime reading – Everything has to be paid for

Many years ago, a legend tells us, a wise old king summoned his advisors to give them a special task.

They were to compile a work containing "the wisdom of the ages". It should serve as an inspiration to all future generations.

It took a long time to complete the task but finally the adviser were able to present the King with the results of their efforts, spanning twelve huge volumes.

This is the wisdom of the ages!" they proclaimed triumphantly to the King.

The King thanked the authors for their tremendous amount of work.
But he was not satisfied. It was much too long. He feared no one would ever read it. He asked his wise men to return to their chambers and condense the volumes.

Eventually, after much consideration and debate, they returned to the King with a single book. He still was not content.

Even this was too long.

The wise men were asked to reduce it even further.

From one volume to one chapter,
From one chapter to one page,
From one page to a single sentence.

At last the King was happy. Once people realize the truth, most of their problems will be solved. Concise and to the point, it reads

"Nothing is for nothing!"

CHAPTER SEVEN -

THE COMMON THREAD THAT PULLS IT ALL TOGETHER

Following our patterns

The aim of this book is to take you through the obstacle course of mental health training to prepare you for the biggest transition in your life. You are going to have to be "fit" in all areas of your health and being tired as you get to the end of your pregnancy is detrimental to the start of your journey into motherhood. Reduce your risks by maximizing the time of your pregnancy to look after yourself and your baby. Sleep when you can, eat the best foods you can afford and engage in regular gentle exercise.

Our next section will look at containment, or how you hold it all together. We will learn to safely use our slipstitch to sit with fear and excitement. We will deconstruct or unpick what might be causing you to be fearful around pregnancy and birth, so that through confronting it, you can understand your fears and reduce their power – or even come to embrace them!

Journal Activity

Keep your journal up to date to record your story for baby and for you. It really doesn't take long; before you will be looking back at this point in time with fondness at your innocence. Enjoy it; it is a magical time, when your body is so busy creating a unique human being inside you. This little person needs you to be available to your process, for everybody's sake.

Relax and enjoy the journey, this really is a one-off trip. No pregnancy is the same and that is one of the reasons why it is so special. Owning and understanding your pregnancy will give you a sense of confidence.

Motherhood

Motherhood is a very complex thing to describe and can be defined as the "art of kinship relation between an offspring and mother, placed in the context of family defined by the qualities characteristic of this relationship." Because of the complexity and differences of a mother's social, cultural and religious roles, beliefs and values, it is challenging to specify a universally acceptable definition for the term "motherhood", but the term itself emphasizes the uniqueness of each individual relationship.

The mantle of motherhood as a concept

The metaphor "mantle of motherhood" allows us to explore ways of looking at the change, responsibility and complex relationships that result from the event of pregnancy and birth. A description or symbol of a mantle allows us to externalize this process from ourselves. We can explore ways of stylizing or wearing the mantle to empower us.

I am curious to see how you might wear this mantle as camouflage, armour, support or comfort. The fabric of the mantle can be examined, washed, coloured, cut and re-styled to suit the needs of the wearer, who may choose to adapt the garment herself, or seek many forms of professional assistance with this task.

The garment, or responsibility, can be worn in an assortment of ways, tightly fitting as a corset for support, or a loose and cosy wrap for comfort and may even be shared between family and friends. It can also be put safely down from time to time. Snags and holes can be repaired, and patches added to overly worn places.

Your values and beliefs inherited from your own mother will be reflected as the mantle is passed from generation to generation onto your shoulders, as it is you who becomes the mother.

Many women that I have worked with have expressed their wish for a more intimate knowledge of motherhood, not the stylized perfection that is too often portrayed in marketing and media. The "rite of passage" that is "motherhood" involves accepting the responsibility of the mantle as it is handed to you, through family values, and beliefs, but also cutting the cloth and sewing the fabric to your own physical capabilities, financial

responsibilities and current social
discourses.

The thread that holds it all together

The thread is a representation of all things that have gone before us in our history. Genetic imprints, family history and values are woven and stitched together to make up our life. List any important information that you are aware of in this area. Below is an example of what I took into my second pregnancy:

My example

Genetics – Mine - Family history of heart disease, cancer, smoking,

My partners *– Family history of cancer, heart disease, alcohol*

Cellular – Mine *– very healthy at the time of pregnancy*

My partners *- Very healthy at the time of pregnancy*

Values – Mine *– Celtic, strong family ties, women are the nurturers, men   are the providers. Strong history of cot deaths in my family – very protective.*

My partners *–Women are strong, nurturing should be shared.*

In my example, you can see that we have conflicting interests in our family values. With hindsight, I can see that this affected the course of my marriage dramatically as events in our lives played out. Ultimately, our differences proved stronger than our similarities. One strand in our thread snapped, and that was enough over time to unravel the fabric of our garment. The results though, are that we have created two beautiful children that are an asset to the world.

The fabric or state of the mantle

The cloth that I inherited through my family values was that pregnancy and birth was a natural healthy process, yet the contradiction exists for me, because my mother had a caesarean section with me and also lost my sisters, one older, one younger, through cot deaths. Thus, I was born into a place of grief, fear and pain. This is my "knowing" and one of my core motivators

Traditionally, mantles are passed on through generations. In biblical terms, 1 Kings 19:19 describes the story of Elijah the prophet passing his mantle of responsibility onto the shoulders of Elasha, who accepted its weight.

The growing cyclic pattern of high intervention and preterm birth in our community means that this knowledge is becoming more commonplace. Meeting the fabric of the mantle through their mothers' birth stories about their own births may set up a pattern of ideas or beliefs around this knowledge, which may be helpful in coping with the experience of the birth of their own children, and influence their style of adaption.

The cutting of the cloth or primary stress episode

High intervention births are proven to increase mortality outcomes for women and their babies. Knowing birth has implications for all involved in its unique transformational process, none more so than the mother, whose cloth is cut, or torn to shape depending on external circumstances. Words for such distressing events are often inadequate in description, for the trauma experienced by the psyche and the soul but the effect is evident at the physical and emotional level.

My example

When my mother gave birth to me she was in an unhappy place. She had lost my sister Katherine in a cot death, was dealing with issues in her marriage and was pressured to conform to the strict values of the Catholic religion in a small country town. She was challenged by her circumstances and thus I was born into grief.

I believe these events have shaped my life. Like Luna Lovegrove in the *Harry Potter* series, I developed the skill of seeing "Thestrals", the black winged horses that pull the coaches to Hogwarts every year. I have an awareness of the effects of pain and loss, and draw on this sensitivity to be helpful. I know it exists and can accept it.

It has shaped me because I am a survivor, a narrative strengthened by the subsequent loss of my second sister Patricia, who also died from cot death. Events play out in my life again and again, but I hold this knowledge as privileged in my psyche and it is helpful to me.

The commitment of my mother's love for me has empowered me to live a full and meaningful life. It is not about perfection or superficialities. My story is about resilience, resourcefulness and reframing for the positive. As research supports, people who are undergoing stress and trauma should not focus on the negative but frame their mindset around a positive, hopeful approach.

Our modern culturally constructed identities are challenging the boundaries of past social constraints. Women's roles have expanded and are in stride with the postmodern concept of the individual with multiple identity variations. We recognize that our view of the world can swing, like a pendulum between opposing points of view due to the many conflicting values we have been exposed to.

Journal Activity

Your reflections

What circumstances were you born into? How did this affect you?
What have you learnt that can be helpful to you now?
Are you still on the same path or has your pendulum swung in another direction?

Do you over compensate in some areas and ignore other aspects of your pregnancy?
How can you create more balance in your approach?

Building a practice of resilience
A narrative metaphor for the running stitch

A running stitch is where the needle is past in and out of the fabric in a consistent fashion to hold two or more pieces of cloth together. It is the most basic of stitches. More thread is visible on the outside of the cloth, than on the underside.

Ground can be covered using this stitch but it has little strength or resiliency. It is often used for tacking and fitting a garment, and can be used as a metaphor for how we run our lives.

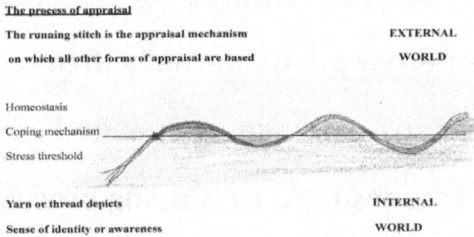

The process of appraisal
The running stitch is the appraisal mechanism
on which all other forms of appraisal are based

EXTERNAL
WORLD

Homeostasis
Coping mechanism
Stress threshold

Yarn or thread depicts
Sense of identity or awareness

INTERNAL
WORLD

Figure 1: The process of appraisal

The running stitch can be used as a metaphor to describe the process of self in appraisal of events passing through the landscape of action, or external world and the landscape of identity, our internal worlds. We assess whether certain stressors are irrelevant, benign or stressful. This is described as the primary appraisal. Secondary appraisal occurs when individuals evaluate, if they can eliminate the stress. If you perceive that effective coping responses are available, both externally and internally then the event or stressor is short-circuited and no stress response occurs. Coping processes can operate as cyclic phases of "retreat' and "encounter". The running stitch metaphor depicts this evaluation as a smooth continuation of the stitch, with much of the assessor's energies and perceptions engaged in the outside world with constructive activities of daily living. The practicalities of the running stitch will hold the event together, but it does not add strength or resiliency

The slip stitch gives strength to the process of bonding

A threat is recognised but not perceived as a threat to

The individual as they believe they have access to resources   **EXTERNAL**

For coping   **WORLD**

Homeostasis

Coping mechanism

Stress threshold   **INTERNAL**

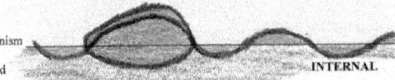

    holds the problem securely in place until   **WORLD**

    the problem can be accommodated

    in a safe isolating space so that normal   **Yarn or thread depicts**

    functioning can continue   **sense of identity or awareness**

Traumatic event or 'going loopy'   **EXTERNAL**

redirects awareness to loop around **WORLD**

event to hold symptoms of the trauma

that occur

- Numbing
- intrusive memories
- Flash backs
- Hypervigilance **INTERNAL**

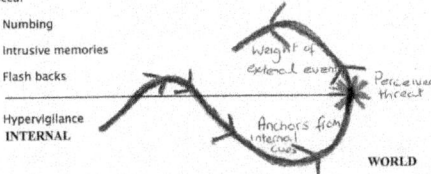

Weight of external event

Perceived threat

Anchors from internal cues

WORLD

Re-looping of awareness until 'security' or 'haemostasis' is re established

The slip stitch

The slip stitch – to move, pass or go smoothly or easily through, a single loop of thread or yarn in the textile arts.

Following on from the running stitch, the slip stitch occurs at the time of the secondary appraisal in the primary stress episode and secondary stress episode if there are enough perceived resources for coping – resiliency is present. The thread or yarn is "looped" back onto itself. If one perceives that effective coping responses are available, then the event or stressor is short-circuited and no stress response occurs. This metaphorical sewing stitch acts to anchor the event in the landscape of identity, keeping it 'safe' for subsequent reappraisal and internalised understanding of strength, coping and hope.

Stress will be experienced if the appraisal is deemed threatening, or the person perceives they do not have sufficient coping strategies. The thread of consciousness continues to loop around on itself, reliving the event in unwanted flashbacks, intrusive thoughts and memories, creating disempowering self-talk, numbing, or hypervigilant experiences or sensations within the body.

Tangle

Traumatic event tangle or knot

- To mix together or intertwine in a   **EXTERNAL**

  Confused mass   **WORLD**

- To catch or hold onto as in a knot
- To enter into an argument
- A state of bewilderment

Homeostasis

Coping mechanism

Stress threshold

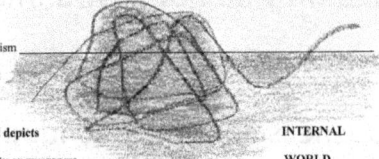

Yarn or thread depicts   **INTERNAL**

Sense of identity or awareness   **WORLD**

Self-ruminating, going round in circles trying to work out an event where assistance is
normally needed to "unpick" a tangle because the event is perceived as too stressful and too
much for the coping resources available

The traumatic event or knot

Uncertainty about your ability to handle a

difficult situation produces stress. It is

important to note that the process of

evaluating the demands of a situation and one's ability to cope occurs at the onset of a stressful event and continues through its duration.

This unrefined "looping around" of consciousness on the event creates a tangled mess, which may require equipment or assistance to "unpick" or deconstruct.

The ideal supports create slip stitches instead of knots and tangles. Appropriate and timely intervention through professional and peer relationships can mitigate the effects of the crisis.

In Summary

A metaphor is a safe way to explore why you do what you do. The mantle of motherhood allows us to access information that we might not otherwise consider important in our pregnancy process. Once aware of a situation that you might not otherwise look at, you can seek assistance in different aspects of your pregnancy.

CHAPTER EIGHT –

APPLY WHAT YOU'VE LEARNED

We have made it through to the end of this journey, but your real journey is just about to begin. This information will support you through all the stages in parenting.

What do you have in your tool kit?

It is standard practice in any pursuit to organize your values and beliefs into a vision. Most corporations have a vision and mission statement, which we have completed for your pregnancy in your journal, which will help clarify your own values and beliefs. Let's review what you

are bringing into your pregnancy. My
mission statement is:

Vision

Privileging the voice of pregnancy, birth
and transition to motherhood by
honouring the values of the individual
mother and the accepted discourse
within our society of a Best Birth
outcome.

Mission Statement
Provide support to give women an
insightful guide to their own values and
beliefs, how these affect their identity,

and can impact on the story of their family.

Assist in acceptance of the reality of their story, through timely intervention, holding the space of motherhood as sancta sanctorum.

Working as an interface to support the existing structure of conception, pregnancy, birth and transition to motherhood.

Work in individual and group session, in person, online and in books to give access to all women in urban and rural community settings

Develop a "new bible" on birthing that is congruent with the changes in contemporary society for women as they transition into "motherhood"

I have embraced my own teachings in the writing of this book, and in the process I am giving birth to ideas and concepts which will be helpful to you. Compile your own book of pregnancy, in the form of your journal. Keep it as a treasure to pass onto your children. Never hesitate to harness the knowledge of your life experience. Preserve it for your future generations. This story will be like gold to you grandchildren and their grandchildren in our consumable and disposable society. It will be fertilizer for their roots.

And remember you are not alone in your journey; every woman who is a mother has made this journey before you, some more successfully than others, but we all get there in the end. This is not a competition. Give yourself a head start though, and do your preparation in good time. Use pregnancy for its purpose, to make you ready to become a mother. Take your time. Enjoy the process and use all the resources you have at your fingertips, as a contemporary, busy woman.

Mental strengths

Run through your checklist of mental strengths. I have listed a few of my favorites below from my own tool kit.

Courage is acting in spite of fear, when the adrenaline is coursing through you veins, knowing you have a center of calm to return to. Develop a practice of working from your center. Rely on your inner guidance. Understand that much of what you fear about pregnancy and birth originates from your subconscious and is not necessarily valid. Nevertheless, listen to these stress impulses and make them your friend. Work with the fear, and move with it. It will hold, support and guide you.

The only requirement for an action to become courageous is to know it's the right thing to do and you wished it was easier. Before you can believe in yourself you have to believe yourself. Practice working outside your comfort zone on a regular basis, breaking your fears down into bit-size pieces, and commit to do whatever it takes to have a best birth outcome for you and your baby.

Balance

Start each day with the intention to be balanced. Work out the priorities in your life by assessing your identities and seeing what can be adapted to adjust to your new role. Balance and peace of mind come from what we have, not what we are missing. Look at the whole, and remember the sliding scale of perspective. Nothing is permanent, be open to change. It is normal to oscillate between two conflicting values.

Health and feelings are affected by energies in your environment. Be selective about where you take your body, stay away from people and places that drain you. Give yourself-permission to shine. Develop and trust your intuition. Embrace the unexpected.

It is necessary to fail in order to learn, and as we learn, we grow. Call them experiences or stepping-stones. You will experience shut downs as your injured self-esteem retreats for recovery from painful or embarrassing situations. Yet the act of failure actually sets you free. As you fail or things don't go as desired, you know you'll live through it, and the pressure is eased. Accept yourself and after a period of rest and retreat you can again embrace your hopes and dreams and get on with your life again.

You will need a team of supportive people to help you. Identify those who can and want to help you. This is no time to be a loner. Bring others into your life that can be on your side. Choose people who recognize your potential and offer encouragement. Moreover, don't be ageist. There is much wisdom and knowledge in older people who have already lived through a lot. They will appreciate being sought after for advice. Don't assume you know it all. Pregnancy is an intricate and complex time. Give yourself time and relax. To benefit from support, you have to be in a place where you can receive it.

Declare an intention to attract helpful people into your life, and let go of those who aren't. Drop competition and the mean team. You may feel particularly vulnerable to judgment, so stay away from it if you can.

Listen to what people want to tell you. There are always gems of wisdom to be obtained in their advice. But remember that they are speaking from their point of view. It is not an essential truth, and it may not be applicable to you. Filter it through attentive ears, see if it fits your view and accept or reject it as you see fit.

Human beings are hard wired to care for pregnant women in their community. Strangers will approach you, to add, assist or annoy, depending on events. Stay calm and centered. Understand that it is a deeply ingrained response on their part, and they probably aren't aware that they are intruding. Set your boundaries gently but firmly. Be comfortable giving back presents you don't want.

Remember, you won't be pregnant forever. It is a short fleeting stage that can feel like an eternity, especially as you grow eager to meet your baby. Talk and connect with your baby constantly throughout your day. Describe where you are going, what you are doing and what you are thinking about out loud. The baby will respond to your voice and know you, your partner and all the important people in your life. The reward will be when you look into your baby's eyes for the first time and you recognize each other.

Positions & Movement

This is a really important aspect of your pregnancy and will be covered fully in my next book. In the meantime, stay in your body, and do appropriate levels of exercise that you enjoy, but don't overdo it. You need strong arms and legs, a healthy back, and you need to be able to breath.

There are many experienced teachers out there who specialize in working with pregnant women. This is not a good time to experiment with a "hard' class or form of exercise. Your body is being amazingly busy twenty-four hours a day. You just won't get to see the results of your hard work for a little while yet.

Find a class that is convenient for you to get to, and attend regularly. You will be surprised by the number of people that purchase attendance to a course and then don't follow through with it. Well-being is not something that can be purchased. It must be worked for and is worth pursuing.

If you can't get to a class start practicing at home. I have compiled a list of asanas that are safe and extremely beneficial for you. Remember, no one else is going to reap the rewards of your practice. This is all for you and your baby.

Shoulder rolls and gentle neck exercises:
Marjariasana (cat yoga pose)
Vajrasana (seated kneeling pose)
Tadasana (mountain pose)
Trikonasana (Triangle yoga posture)

Veerbhadrasana (warrior yoga posture)

Supported Paschimottanasana (seated forward bend)

Titliasana (gentle butterfly yoga posture)

Viptritkarni (against the wall)

Shavasana/ Yoga Nidra

Acupuncture for pregnancy

Acupuncture is now an accepted form of treating the bodies energy systems. Your practitioner will take a full history, check your pulses and observe you tongue to see where the energy is stuck, or running to weakly.

They will then insert tiny, hygienic safety needles to move or stimulate the energy through your meridian system. This stimulates the healthy flow of chi, alleviating symptoms and promoting your body's ability to heal itself.

Your therapist will work with your energy to help and support the growth of your baby.

Mood setting

Setting your mood to stay connected to your baby is really important. There are many things that you can do that work for you. Lighting and music are important forms of relaxation and your baby will respond and enjoy them. You will soon understand when your baby doesn't share your taste in music, movement or food. Don't ignore this information. It is the beginning of your relationship and baby needs to know you are willing to respond to its needs too.

Relaxation & Visualization

Visualizing your birth during your pregnancy will help you to become more comfortable with the process when labour does arrive. Whether you have a vaginal delivery, or a caesarean birth, you have followed your baby. This is your job in labour, to follow your baby, adjusting to the labour process. Allow yourself to move out of the way and let the process be.

If your labour takes you down a different path from your expectations, you will find the metaphors from your bedtime reading useful in dealing with change. The suggestions given will help you to adjust in a more relaxed manner to whatever situation comes up. Greater resources for adaptation will be available to you, as you put to rest other distractions that might otherwise be present in your family history.

Address your unique concerns about family adjustment and birth history with your doctor or midwife and trusted friends. This personalized experience will allow you to work through feelings associated with childbirth before delivery, thereby reducing tension and fear during labour. Find a suitable prenatal support class in your area, the time and money invested is invaluable to your process and understanding.

Meditation & Intuition

Intuition emerges best when we are relaxed and receptive. Allowing the deeper parts of ourself to connect with our conscious processes. When we live in fear or worry, it can't come through as easily. Science and sceptics belittle this feminine trait because it is difficult to "prove" how it works or even if it exists.

By developing self reflection you will become more aware of your inner voice and by listening to it develop your ability to relate to your intuition, trust your process and move more confidently through your pregnancy.

The key to increasing intuition is being more relaxed. Get your brain to spend more time in alpha rather than beta mode. Stay calm and open and let go of fear and worry for your best birth outcome.

Emotional Freedom Techniques - EFT

This is a great self-help tool that I regularly use in my classes. EFT is an emotional, needle free version of acupuncture based on the connection between your body's subtle energies, your emotions and your health. EFT involves tapping on the meridian points of traditional Chinese acupuncture whilst focusing on a problem. Most people experience a relaxation response almost immediately, as well as a lessening of the feeling associated with the problem and more positive thinking patterns. It can be learned for free on line.

Neuro Emotional Technique –NET

I am an advanced certified NET practitioner. NET is a mind-body stress-reduction technique that uses a methodology of finding and removing neurological imbalances related to an unresolved mind-body component. NET is a tool that is used by practitioners of all disciplines to help improve behavioural and physical conditions. NET is a Mind-Body stress relief technique that has generated an incredible amount of excitement since 1988 and is very effective.

Hypnosis

Self-hypnosis or hypnosis performed by working with a practitioner, such as a hypno-birthing expert in their childbirth education program, may be helpful for teaching relaxation and techniques that will encourage you and your baby to connect.

Talking With the Baby

I can't emphasis this enough. It is free, effective and beautiful. Talk to your baby and let the baby know that they are loved, wanted and cared for. Dad can talk to the baby too, on the belly and close to the skin.

Diet

It is important to eat well. The Australian Dietary Guidelines recommend that you:

Eat plenty of vegetables, legumes (such as chickpeas and lentils) and fruits

Eat plenty of cereals (including breads, rice, pasta and noodles), preferably wholegrain. Include lean meat, fish, poultry and/or alternatives. Also include milks, yoghurts, cheeses and/or alternatives. It is recommended that you choose reduced-fat varieties where possible.

Drink plenty of water. Drinking more water increases the volume of amniotic fluid in which your baby thrives. Keep in mind that too much fluid can also be problematic and you need to consult with your doctor if you get swollen ankles or shortness of breath.

Limit saturated fat and moderate total fat intake. Choose foods low in salt. Eat only moderate amounts of sugars and foods containing added sugars.

Your body becomes more efficient when you're expecting a baby and makes even better use of the energy you obtain from the food you eat. Following the old saying "eating for two" is not necessary. Your appetite is your best guide of how much food you need to eat. You may find your appetite fluctuates throughout your pregnancy.

In the first few weeks your appetite may fall away dramatically and you may not feel like eating proper meals, especially if you have been feeling sick. During the middle part of your pregnancy, your appetite may be the same as before you became pregnant or slightly increased. Towards the end of your pregnancy your appetite will probably increase. It is important to have small frequent meals at this time. Your baby takes up so much space; large meals are no longer tolerable, as they can't be squeezed into the limited space.

The best rule to remember is to eat when you are hungry.

Massage & Aromatherapy

The act of massage can be very relaxing in itself. While you're pregnant, having your feet, shoulders, or tummy gently massaged with lovely-smelling oil can feel wonderful.

However, it doesn't work for everyone. Pregnancy can make your skin tight, dry and sensitive, and being touched may not relax you at all. Also, some essential oils may make you itch, so tell your therapist if you develop itchy skin after having a treatment.

You can try using essential oils in a compress, too. You can make a compress by adding a couple of drops of oil into 250ml of warm water. Soak a flannel in the water and place it on the small of your back, your forehead, or your tummy to help relax you.

The chemicals within some oils are also thought to improve your general well-being. Essential oils such as common lavender, chamomile, or ylangylang are considered safe during pregnancy.

Homeopathy

Homeopathic medicines will help improve your health as well as your baby's. They are gentle, safe, non-toxic, and approved and effective in treating various common problems of pregnancy and childbirth. However you are advised to seek out a qualified and experienced practitioner for your pregnancy.

Chiropractor

Chiropractic care is health maintenance of the spinal column, discs, related nerves and bones without drugs or surgery. It involves adjusting misaligned joints of the body, especially of the spine, which reduces spinal nerve stress and therefore promotes health throughout the body.

There are no known contraindications to chiropractic care throughout pregnancy and many recorded benefits. The nervous system is the master communication system to all the body systems including the reproductive system. Keeping the spine aligned helps the entire body work more effectively.

Doctor or midwife

Choosing an attending doctor or midwife for your birth is a big decision. One of the best ways to start is to know what sort of birth you want.

Then decide where you want to give birth. If you set for a home birth, then your decision will be easier, as only independent midwives attend to these births. However, if you are going to have a hospital birth, you may want to reflect on the type of establishment you choose and the services that they offer.

An experienced team of doctors, nurses and midwives runs the obstetric unit of your local community hospital. If you require more support you will be referred to a larger teaching hospital where they specialize in high intervention births and support of preterm or sick babies. These are big institutions that may feel busy and impersonal, but offer specialized care.

Many hospitals offer a more informal birthing unit, where the environment is less clinical, but emergency medical assistance is available if you require it. Take your time in deciding where you want to birth; ask to look around the facilities. Many routinely offer a tour and consult with as many practitioners as you need to make a decision.

Talk to your care provider about any concerns that you have. You have behaved responsibly to yourself and your baby if you have voiced your concerns. Choose a caregiver that you can relate to. Communication plays a major part in your experience of birth.

The experience of birth and life is a complex and intricate process. Being pregnant places you at the forefront of the experience of life. Like a tree growing from its roots through its farthest branches, we experience life in pregnancy as though we are at the very tip of the branches, reaching out to what we want;

family, connection, intimacy, growth and love. Yet when do this we are branching into unknown and unstructured space. Trust your roots for nourishment and your branches for support. Create and sow together the life that you want for your family, and start at the beginning with solid foundations of knowing your pregnancy, for yourself, your partner, your children and your grandchildren. Leave your mark, and your inheritance as knowledge of your pattern on your fabric of consciousness that is your mantle. As worn by the women that went before you, and the women that will come in future generations. Don't dismiss its value

to you or to them. Privilege it, for it is
your self-worth.

Relaxation
Technique
click hear to listen
and enjoy

Bedtime reading – "Shine your light" Written by Marianne Williamson in "A return to Love"

Our deepest fear is not that we are

inadequate.

Our deepest fear is that we are powerful

beyond measure.

It is our light not our darkness that most

frightens us.

We ask ourselves "who am I to be

brilliant, gorgeous, talented, fabulous?"

You are a child of the Goddess.

Your playing small doesn't serve the world.

There's nothing enlightened about shrinking

So that other people don't feel insecure around you.

We are all meant to shine, like children do.

We were born to make manifest the glory of the Goddess that is within us.

It's not just in some of us: it's in everyone.

And as we let our own light shine,

We unconsciously give other people permission to do the same.

As we're liberated from our own fear,
Our presence automatically liberates others.

CHAPTER NINE -

TAKING THE STRESS OUT OF PREGNANCY AND BIRTH

Stress Reduction

Slow down

If there is one thing that you can do during your pregnancy, it is to slow down. This will happen to you sooner or later so make a conscious practice of it at the start of your pregnancy.

Regular relaxation is a crucial part of slowing down. Our hurried pace has become so much a part of our daily existence that it even seems to manifest in the air we breathe, but we are not genetically coded to rush constantly and such rushing can affect your growing babies. "Hurry up" is an injunction that many of us have embodied from a very early age. Even when there are no external demands on us, there is an internal feeling to occupy our time with doing something productive.

Your body is being productive twenty-four hours a day. You have planted a seed of life deep inside you. Give it time, your love and be patient with the process. This is just the beginning.

It is up to you to decide whether you want to slow down and relax. Reassure yourself that it is OK to stop, take your time, breath, sit down and think about what you want and need. The underlying message is that your pregnancy is important to you, more than anybody else.

Get organized

Focus your attention and organize yourself. Practice the tasks in this book to help you sort out your priorities and responsibilities. Write lists. Get the information out of your head and onto paper. This has a calming effect on the nervous system.

Prioritize your lists. Today, this week, this month, this pregnancy. Ask yourself "Is it really important? Who has made that decision and why? Will you feel just as happy, safe content if you let it go? Is it real? Is it really real?"

Treat yourself with respect. Constantly flogging yourself to do more and more is a form of subtle self-abuse. Be respectful to those around you; don't expect the world to change just because you are going to. Take the pressure off wherever you can as no one is perfect, and nothing real is picture perfect as depicted by media and marketing campaigns. They want your money, not your happiness.

Slow down, organize yourself and choose where you spend your time wisely. Your investment in your pregnancy will come back to you many times over.

Stay with the activities that make your heart sing, nourish your body with good food and exercise regularly. Nourish your mind too. What goes into you through your senses becomes part of who you are and what your baby will become. Use your slower pace to pay attention to the beauty in the world through your senses.

Find inspiring books, articles and friends. Research ways on how to live and to be that suit your values and inspire you. Spend time with like-minded people. Fun and laughter are an important part of relaxing and rejuvenating yourself. Don't just do something, sit still and chill.

Remember the bigger picture

There will be many things to attend to during your pregnancy, but the most important for reducing your stress is your attitude and awareness. Developing this require responsibility and commitment on your part. You are building up the mental strength to take care of yourself, your baby and your family, the mantle has been passed onto your shoulders.

Reflect on its beauty and its love. Keep it real, persevere and treasure it.

Stop trying to do more than one thing at a time. You will develop the ability to concentrate and this skill will help your composure. Cultivate a sense of self assurance, even under fire, by focusing your attention on the moment. Focus on what you want, complete as much as you can then move onto the next thing. Bring patience and attentiveness to your pregnancy. If your attention gets stuck in a repetitive problem in your mind,move your body, breathe and choose a task that demands your full concentration. Especially if it's in the middle of the night!

Get up and make yourself a cup of tea, focus on your breathing and send love to your baby. It will be a while before you sleep well again. But it will be worth the effort. In the beginning you will have to work on this journey, but persevere, as your children grow your efforts will be feed back to you a thousand fold. Enjoy.

Centering
Techneque

Notes

Notes

Notes

Notes
Notes
Notes

Notes

Notes

BIBLIOGRAPHY

A Book of Comfort, Dr R Brasch
The Circles, Kerry Armstrong
Shopping for a Shrink, Todd Zemek
Echoes of the Early Tides, Tony Moore
The FetalMatrix, P Gluckman& M Hanson
Maps of Narrative Practice, Michael White
Natural Brilliance, Paul Scheele
Reaching for the Stars, Margot Cairnes
What is Narrative Therapy?, Alice Morgan